ADVANCE

CHAKRA

HEALING

———

Heart Disease

ADVANCED

CHAKRA

HEALING

The Four Pathways Approach

HEART DISEASE

Cyndi Dale

CROSSING PRESS
Berkeley I Toronto

CROSSING PRESS

an imprint of Ten Speed Press
P.O. Box 7123
Berkeley, California 94707
www.tenspeed.com

Distributed in Australia by Simon and Schuster Australia,
in Canada by Ten Speed Press Canada, in New Zealand
by Southern Publishers Group, in South Africa by Real Books, and in the
United Kingdom and Europe by Publishers Group UK.

Cover and text design by Lisa Buckley Design, San Francisco, CA
Typesetting by Tasha Hall

Library of Congress Cataloging-in-Publication Data

Dale, Cyndi.
  Advanced Chakra healing : heart disease : the four pathways approach
/ by Cyndi Dale.
    p. cm.
  Includes bibliographical references and index.
  ISBN-13: 978-1-58091-171-9
  ISBN-10: 1-58091-171-4
  1. Heart—Diseases—Alternative treatment—Popular works.
2. Chakras—Health aspects—Popular works. I. Title.
  RC684.A48D35 2007
  616.1'206—dc22
2006034148

Disclaimer: The author fully recognizes and accepts the value of the
traditional medical profession. The ideas, suggestions, and healing techniques
in this book are not intended as a substitute for proper medical attention.
Any application of these ideas, suggestions, and techniques is
at the reader's sole discretion.

Printed in the United States of America
1 2 3 4 5 6 7 8 9 10 — 11 10 09 08 07

Contents

Acknowledgments

There are so many people who have touched my heart that I feel I am one of the luckiest people on this planet. Foremost, I want to acknowledge Wendy Kardia, my friend and business organizer, whose last name means heart and describes her perfectly. For daily inspiration that is heartfelt (and entirely too honest), my thanks to friends J. J. Jeska, Cathy Scofield, and a blessing to Carol Lee, who listens with—and lives from—her heart. An ode to Lauren Star, who is as generous as she is brave; and gratitude to Dr. Debra Arone, acupuncturist and healer extraordinaire, who has gently helped to heal both my physical and my spiritual heart.

It takes true heart (and grit) to serve as my editor, which Melissa Moore does with perception and humor. And finally, my deepest gratitude to Jo Ann Deck, publisher of Crossing Press and a woman of courage and grace.

Introduction

When he learned I was writing about heart disease, a Czech friend of mine sent me a book titled *A Nail Merchant at Nightfall*. I looked at the dusty old text and wondered what it had to do with heart disease. I opened to this passage:

> "In this way I happened to ransack my wife's linen cupboard as well, and of course I did not find my lost tax bill there; instead, to my surprise, under the linen I found my heart, which apparently she had tucked away in some absent-minded moment, leaving it hidden and forgotten for years under the linen."[1]

The passage speaks to what I believe is the root of heart disease. All over the world, our hearts are in trouble. We have individually and collectively misplaced them and made them sick. To heal your heart, you must first find it. This book will show you how. Through the healing of your heart, you can then begin to live from the heart, from the source of your inner dreams and wisdom.

Advanced Chakra Healing: Heart Disease supports traditional and medically recognized methods for healing heart disease. At one level, almost all heart problems originate in bodily causes, such as genetic abnormalities, viral infections, poor diet, and bad habits like smoking. It's imperative to address heart problems with practical and physical methods. This perspective will take you only to the first gate of healing, however. There is always more to healing a heart condition than analysis and treatment for specific physical stresses. Physical treatment is only the first of four roads that make up the treatment of the heart.

These roads are called the pathways. These pathways are, in fact, four different levels of awareness. Travel any of these thoroughfares and you reach the same destination—the place you want to be. Your goal? The healed self, who exists already in the Greater Reality, a space in which we experience heaven and Earth as the same.

In the Greater Reality, your heart is already healed because you know yourself as unconditionally loved and loving. There is no need for heart trouble because your heart cannot be troubled.

Love, you see, is always the key to healing the heart. This is an easy statement to make, but not always an easy truth to understand.

Reading this book is like unfolding a map. You begin wherever you are. Your final destination is healing. Healing is not the same as curing. To cure is to become free of symptoms and the physical manifestation of a disorder. To heal means to make whole; to recognize that in the Greater Reality, you are already whole, and therefore healed. You might release the emotions causing heart pain and still need surgery for the remaining physical disorder. You might enjoy an instantaneous cleansing of plaque and still have a need to feel your long-held feelings.

The four approaches to healing include but also transcend the limited options offered through traditional or alternative care. You can journey any or all of these pathways to find and heal your heart. What works for you? Take out your map and see.

Tour along the *elemental pathway* and you devote yourself to issues physical, emotional, or mental in nature. Trek on the *power pathway* and you'll be supercharged with forces that can only be called supernatural. Voyage on the *imagination pathway* and you invite forth your magical self, the one who can create with a thought, a word, and a need. Slip onto the *divine pathway* and you find yourself in the heart of the Divine, who has been holding your heart dearly oh, so many years. Each of these pathways presents an entirely valid and real way to heal from heart disease, for you exist on each pathway simultaneously, just as you already reside in the Greater Reality, whole and healed.

I first introduced the Four Pathways system in my guidebook, *Advanced Chakra Healing*. This process is adaptable to any disease or problem. I have shown people how to apply its principles to healing from cancer in *Advanced Chakra Healing: Cancer*. I am now particularly grateful to adapt the concepts to the heart, as I have struggled with a heart problem for years and have the Four Pathways to thank for my current level of health.

You can traverse any one or all four of these pathways to transform a heart condition into a healed state. Which highway or byway to travel is your decision and will depend upon your personality. Each pathway presents healing via a unique "key," or set of codes, clues, and techniques. For any pathway, you will determine your game plan by using your *intuition*, your inner guidance that receives input from the Divine. To conduct diagnosis and healing, to transfer knowledge or energies from one pathway to another, and to leap from pathway to pathway, you utilize yet another universal tool, the chakras.

Chakras are an ancient and mystical set of energy organs and, as such, are part of a larger structure called the human energy system. The *human energy system* is a set of fast- and slow-moving organs that can transfer information, disease, and problems out of the body and transport healing and healthy information into the body. By working with the energy underneath your heart disease, you can quickly effect change and healing. I use the term *energy mapping* to describe the actual process used in the Four Pathways program: map the desired change, chart your course, pinpoint the energies causing your problem, and you shift those energies for health and wellness.

I use a twelve-chakra healing system, concentrating on the first eleven for most healing work. If you are already familiar with the concept of chakras, you will know that many experts propose a seven- or perhaps eight-chakra system. Almost all practitioners acknowledge the existence of many other secondary chakras, for the human body is full of energy bodies that support our physical and spiritual well-being. Gifted with psychic sight since I was a child, I have perceived and worked with chakras atop the basic seven since I was young. I suggest you employ the additional chakras, because healing is phenomenally increased with their use. These additional chakras tap into forces and powers that can magnetize universal energies to greatly boost your healing capacity.

I also use phrases such as *heart disease, heart trouble, heart condition,* and the like interchangeably, all to reference the broader term, cardiovascular disease. *Cardiovascular disease* is a general term for a collection of diseases and conditions; it is not actually a disease itself. It refers to any condition or disease that adversely affects your cardiovascular system, which is composed of your heart (cardio) and all your blood vessels (vascular). Although it's not medically correct to use a phrase like *heart disease* interchangeably with *cardiovascular disease*, I do so for two reasons. First, comfort. Most of us use these terms interchangeably. Second, energetic accuracy. All cardiovascular diseases have some involvement with the fourth chakra, known as the heart chakra.

In this book, you'll learn how to shift heal. *Shift healing* involves moving energies inside of or among any of the four pathways so you can heal from heart disease. Mastering this process is dependent upon accepting your role as your own healer. To be effective, you need a working knowledge of the tools in your Four Pathways medical bag. Your generic instruments can be used on any pathway. These include your own intuition, or inner guidance, which is imperative for energy mapping. There are tools unique to each pathway as well. You'll be shown how to recognize and use these in the chapters about each pathway.

Although the Four Pathways approach presents like a map of four different countries, it's important to know that you decide where to journey or not. You can choose among the pathways or stay right where you are! In the Four Pathways system, you set your own course. You can decide whether to heal or not—and even what healing means to you. This self-responsibility is fundamental to the Four Pathways approach, for in this system, you serve as your own healer. You rely on your own intuition to work within your personal energy system to create an energy map for healing. In short, you become your own *shift healer*, shifting diseased energies out and healthy energies in. Accepting this much responsibility can be frightening until you remember that your intuition links you not only with your inner self but also with the Divine. Through your connection with the Divine, you can, at any moment, link through the Greater Reality with anyone and everything else. This world and all worlds beyond it stand ready to assist you in this most marvelous of adventures, the voyage into your own heart!

Your odyssey will be unique to you. This is why I have organized this book so that you can pick and choose which pathway or technique best suits you. In the first half of the book, I introduce the basics of the Four Pathways approach and its application to heart disease. I then provide the fundamental definitions and techniques of the Four Pathways system, including a full chapter on understanding and using your intuition, your major tool for diagnosing and healing. You are now prepared for the second half of the book, which outlines each of the four pathways and a plethora of techniques for practical application. The end of the book isn't the end of your expedition—you may revisit it and the mother guide, *Advanced Chakra Healing*, over and over for inspiration and ideas. In many ways, reaching the finale of the book is the commencement of the grandest quest of all—the full ownership of your Greater Self, the self whose heart beats in time with the heart of God.

I return again to the fundamental question: *Where is your heart?* Did you forget about it? Did you give it to another, and never take it back? Did you think it too vulnerable and lock it behind walls? You have no reason to hide, for you are already the self that you are meant to become. You are you. That is the ultimate beginning—and end—of healing: the place where your heart is.

PART *One*

chapter one

Heart Problems as an Invitation to Love

We are too little to be always able to rise above difficulties. Well, then, let us pass beneath them quite simply.

—St. Thérèse de Lisieux

More people die of heart problems than they do the next seven types of deadly diseases, which include various types of cancer and autoimmune diseases, combined. Whereas one in twenty-seven women will die from breast cancer, one in two will die from heart disease.[1] In fact, one in every four Americans has one or more types of heart disease.[2] What could make your heart, the center of life and love, turn into a ticking time bomb? In the time it could take you to answer, just thirty-three seconds, someone else in the United States will die of heart disease.

Physicians, spiritualists, and poets agree that the heart is your most vital organ. Physicians explain that your heart keeps you alive, pumping blood through thousands of miles of blood vessels. It is the physical center of your circulatory system, the manager of 75 trillion cells. Religious experts stress that the heart is the house of the soul, the placeholder of love and relationship. Personally, I favor the poet's argument, which lyrically points out that all of life's problems originate in the heart, including heartbreaks and heartaches. All this attention on a relatively small organ; the heart is only as large as your fist.

When afflicted with heart disease, it's important to follow the counsel of your physicians. Be practical. To heal fully, however, you must go deeper. A damaged heart is not just an injured organ. It is a wise counselor that will show you how to heal. Your heart fails you only because you are failing to hear its call for love.

A Greater Reality

The Greater Reality is a level of awareness in which everything and everyone is whole. Each of us occupies the Greater Reality, which is a lot like heaven on earth. In this state, we have no heart disease. In this place, we have no problems. We aren't perfect, for perfection isn't necessary for wellness; in fact, perfection stands in opposition to wholeness. Perfection leads to stagnation. If things were perfect, there would be no striving, no growth, no distinction of personalities, and no motivation for love. There would be no need to look into the eyes of a lover, a child, a friend, or an enemy, and bridge one heart to another. There would be no love.

To heal your heart, you must join hands with your physicians as well as the spiritualists and poets. You must acknowledge your heart as a door into the Greater Reality.

Essentially, healing occurs when you tap into your Greater Self, the self who dwells in the Greater Reality, and allow yourself to transform partially into him or her. Most people ignore this reality because they believe the Greater Reality is a just reward for a good life, and they are waiting to die to enjoy it. Why wait until death, when you can receive the blessings of heaven right now? Why not love yourself enough to accept this reality as your only reality?

The source of this magnificent love is available to us all, regardless of our creed, ethnicity, gender, or age. There are many traditional names for this source, including God, Allah, Christ, Buddha, Krishna, and the Mother. Others attribute this power to the inner self, and still others to the wellspring of human faith or connection. It doesn't matter what you call the source, for why would "Love" care what "It" is called? Love only cares that you call upon it!

Love unifies everyone, holding us in good health and happiness. There's a part of each of us that recognizes the truth of love and is in complete agreement about its healing powers. This is the self who exists totally in the Greater Reality. I call this aspect of self your spirit, essence, or Greater Self. Your spirit knows that it is completely and unconditionally loved. It doesn't require an illness or a problem to learn that it is so loved.

Your spiritual self is also smart enough to know that your physical self might require a demonstration of love in order to believe in love. It's okay to have heart disease. Being sick doesn't negate your spiritual beauty, essential beliefs, or inner strength. Being sick means that in human form, you want your heart to remind you of your lovableness. The heart chooses to send these messages in the form of heart disease.

None of us is trained to perceive, acknowledge, or operate within the Greater Reality. We learn how to sharpen pencils and spell words at school, send thank-you cards and e-mails to communicate, dress for success and smile at the boss to make money, and take aspirin or check our pulse at the first sign of a heart irregularity. No one teaches us how to live as a spirit embodied in a physical body. No one teaches us how to summon forth the healed self, the self of the Greater Reality, in order to heal ourselves physically. What is the key to unlocking our Greater Self and hidden powers? We must claim our inherent wholeness, the imperfect human self. All four pathways lead to this recognition.

Energy, the Essence of Healing

Everything in the universe—your dog, your books, your thoughts, your feelings, your heart—is made of energy. *Energy* is the product of information and vibration. For example, imagine that a friend has presented you with two cups of liquid, one cup of tea and the other coffee. What makes these two fluids essentially different? Well, there's some type of information that is telling the tea to be tea and the coffee to be coffee. Everything visible and invisible, concrete and intangible is "informed" by these codes of information.

Now peer into your cup of coffee, down to the molecular and subatomic level, to see what is really brewing. I like to make the analogy that the subatomic world is like a nursery school room of toddlers. Matter never sits still. Everything—every piece and parcel of matter in the universe—vibrates or moves. Coffee atoms move at a different rate or frequency than do tea atoms. The information is responsible for this difference in vibration. If you telescope in further, you'll see that some of the coffee particles aren't even in the cup! There might be a few already in your stomach, a few still hovering in the plant fields, maybe even a couple dancing about in a different world. But that's a discussion for later, when we take the top off of physical reality to look at the quantum world underneath. For now, the essential point is this: everything is made of energy.

Energy is a matter of "informed vibration," the information that tells something how fast and far to move. For our purposes, we can now look at heart disease as involving irregular or unhealthy informed vibration.

Grasping this concept is critical to performing shift healing on the Four Pathways system. What if you could change harmful data on one pathway and make your heart vibrate in a healthier manner? Perhaps you could apply forces from yet another pathway to alter vibration, which in turn tells the "sick information" to be "well information." Seeing your heart as an energy organ is the foundation of true heart healing.

Your Heart as an Energy Organ

Do you think your brain controls your body? Think again. The heart's electromagnetic field (EMF) is five thousand times more powerful than the EMF field created by the brain. Quantitative devices show that the heart emanates fifty thousand femtoteslas (a measure of EMF) in comparison to the ten femtoteslas that emit from the brain.[3] Still other research separates the electrical from the magnetic powers of the brain, showing that, as measured by an electrocardiogram (ECG), the heart's electrical field is sixty times greater in amplitude than the brain's, and its magnetic field is five thousand times stronger.[4]

Your heart just might be the real brain of your body, its rhythms and knowledge ordering your health and wellness. Two new disciplines, cardio-energetics and neurocardiology, suggest this very idea, encouraging people to "mind" their hearts in order to "mind" their bodies. A great deal of research supports the vital role played by the heart in regulating the health of every cell and organ, as well as the overall condition of our bodies.

Perhaps most interesting and accessible is the research generated by the Institute of HeartMath in Boulder Creek, California. According to one of their research booklets, *Science of the Heart*, the heart plays many vital roles that are not taught in science classes.[5] It functions as its own independent neurological center, drawing upon 40,000 neurons to detect circulating hormones and neurochemicals, as well as heart rate and blood pressure information, which is then sent to the brain. The heart generates much of this information from inside of the heart itself (in chapter 5, I suggest that some of this information is psychic or intuitive in nature).

The heart was actually reclassified as a hormone gland in 1983, when scientists determined that it produced atrial natriuretic peptide, a hormone that affects the blood vessels, kidneys, adrenal glands, and brain. The heart also generates oxytocin, a "love hormone" which produces bonding and affection between people, in quantities equal to that made in the brain, reinforcing the age-old belief that the heart is the center of love.

The authors of *Science of the Heart* also state that the heart is the most powerful generator of rhythmic information. Through the patterns of its beat, the heart communicates information relevant to one's emotional state to the medulla, which feeds data to the thalamus and amygdala, which then "speak" to the frontal lobes. This means that the patterns of your heart, created from information gathered inside and outside itself, stimulate stored emotions and beliefs, which in turn tell your brain how to make decisions. You could say that your heart is one of the brains of your body.

As summarized in the booklet *The Energetic Heart*, the heart produces patterns that are neurological, hormonal, and electrical. As recorded in various types of cardiac rhythms, changes in the heart affect every cell in the body. Studies show that data is also recorded between neurological impulses, intervals of pressure, or electromagnetic waves. Even when your heart is "quiet," it is carrying emotional information that affects your conscious perception of feelings—and the world![6]

Certain studies reveal that the heart even carries an imprint of our unique personalities. Consider that people receiving heart transplants eventually take on the characteristics of their heart donors, even to the degree of remembering the donors' memories.[7]

Our hearts hold the events and perceptions of our lives, but they are also intimate to the unfolding of our genetics. Many scientists believe you become what your genes tell you to be, and the way you're raised is a secondary factor in your unfolding. Now there's evidence showing that your genes directly instruct your personalities through vibration and also through the heart.[8] Researchers G. Rein and Rollin McCraty show that DNA, the carriers of your genetic coding, receive and transmit information through your heart's electrical rhythms and their own vibrations.[9] Heart disease may be carried in part in your genes, but by changing the energy of your heart, you might also be able to alter the DNA that causes heart disease. In fact, your heart is structured to affect (and be effected by) your DNA.

The Heart Heals through Energy

If there's one point I want you to grasp from this book, it is this: The heart holds the key to its own healing.

Your heart is an energy organ. It conducts thousands of times more electricity than does the brain. What information should the heart carry in its electrical circuitry? What information—what vibrations—will guarantee health? The heart also generates more magnetic energy than does the brain, creating a magnetic field that radiates several feet away from your body. What messages do you want to send into and receive from the world?

For a moment, imagine there are two realities. There is the reality that you were raised in. This is the world of struggle. This world trains you to believe you have to earn love. You must be good, kind, religious, accept-able, or perfect enough to become worthy of love. But you can never be good enough to earn love because you are human, with all the flaws that implies. You can never meet people worthy of your love, for they, too, are human. In this world, everyone has a heart condition, for our hearts are contracted, perhaps even completely closed. Here, the human heart is dis-eased or ill at ease.

Wrapped within this reality is the Greater Reality, a reality that func-tions in such higher truths as faith, hope, joy, and acceptance. Here, you never wonder whether you are lovable. If you exist, it is because the Divine loves you. Because you exist, you are loved. Because you are loved, you can love. Why question your worthiness—it's not even an issue!

You can transcend into this Greater Reality simply by recognizing its existence. Once we recognize its existence, there are four pathways to help us reach this illuminated state. Just as there are four chambers of the heart, so too there are four levels of awareness that serve to transform your perceptions so that you can see there is only love. Four heart chambers, four pathways. Four paths, one heart.

We begin pathway healing by acknowledging the power of choice. We can choose which reality is our reality. We become healed because of the choices we make—in our hearts.

The New Science of Healing

The Four Pathways process is based on a medley of so-called "New Science" constructs, including quantum physics, chaos theory, general physics, the theory of relativity, sacred geometry, and fractal mathematics. Some general concepts that are found in "New Science" are:

- Matter can move faster and slower than the speed of light.
- You can control where matter moves and in what form it will appear.
- What is concrete can be made intangible, and what is intangible can be made concrete.

There are two basic units of matter: Tachyons, which are subatomic particles that can move faster than the speed of light; and quarks, which move slower than the speed of light. One type of particle can transform into another. Under certain conditions, either one can convert from particle to waveform and back again. Remember that energy is the same as informed vibration. If you can make information move faster than the speed of light, you can shift "bad data" out of your body to a place far, far away, thereby removing a heart problem.

On the other hand, you can also change vibration from fast to slow, bringing "good data" into your body and healing a heart problem. Perhaps your heart has never achieved its "perfect vibration," and now is suffering for it. Perhaps in some other world, what physicists call the antiworld, your heart beats in perfect symmetry. You can transfer this antiworld heart's vibrations from this "idea space," slow it down to quark speed, and bring it into your body, creating a perfectly good heart in the present.

As my brief stories illustrate, what is solid can be made immaterial; what is ethereal can be transformed into the tangible. Shift healing is not only possible, it is also the only type of healing that has ever been performed on this planet. From a scientific point of view, shift healing is about changing either or both information and vibration so you can exchange one reality for another. When a cardiologist lifts out a diseased heart and transplants a healthy one, he or she is conducting shift healing. Hawthorn, an herb used to relax the heart, works neurologically, aiding the body in substituting one set of chemical reactions for another. Meditation assists the brain in changing from an over-stimulated wave pattern to a more peaceful one. When you think good thoughts, you hope to exchange them for bad ones. When you hold happy feelings, you encourage the release of harmful ones. You've been using shift healing your entire life, and you just haven't known it.

Working with the Four Pathways approach provides you more choices and control over your shift healing capabilities. There are different ways of getting energy to change on each pathway, because each pathway manages energy in a different way. But before you can traverse the miraculous worlds of the pathways, you need to know a little bit more about them.

The Four Paths to Greatness

There are four basic pathways, or levels of awareness, and each leads into the Greater Reality, a place where the Greater Self resides, whole and healed. Each is an independent path for heal-ing, available in the blink of an eye. Remember my point about shift healing? You've been doing it your entire life! Well, you've also been walking on each of these four path-ways for just as long, because you already exist upon each of them simultaneously.

Each pathway is unique and has its own functions, operating rules, energy bodies, and healing energies.

You'll probably find yourself more com-fortable with one or maybe two pathways, rather than all four. This is natural. It's still important to have a working knowledge of

The four paths to the Greater Reality are made of physicality, supernaturalism, creative magic, and divine love.

each pathway because of the variety of healing energies and tech-niques available to you. When you're stuck in one plane, you can jump to another for assistance.

To help you understand the pathways, I will illustrate a person from each one. As I do this, think of your own history. What types of experiences can be explained according to pathway differences? Have some fun coming up with your own analogies.

Story One: Joseph Gets Unstuck

For years, Joseph had kept his dilapidated car together on the road with creative repairs as far-flung as chewing gum, paper clips, peppercorns, and hope. His friends couldn't believe his luck, which he attributed to a "good jinn" in the car engine.

One day he and his friends took a road trip to a small town. They took three cars, Joseph driving his. After spending some time in the small town, the friends piled back into Joseph's car and the caravan began heading home—for a while. Joseph's car decided to stop at an intersection—and not budge again.

He tried all sorts of techniques, as did his friends. A believer in his "special magic," Joseph even performed a little dance around the car, attempting to coax it back to life. Nothing worked. Finally, a doctor friend of his said, "Joseph, maybe the car is just plain broken!"

Joseph had the car towed to a nearby station, at which the mechanic confirmed the diagnosis. "You basically have no engine left," he stated. "Your car has broken down." Joseph glowered. He didn't like being so practical, but the reality of the situation could not be denied.

Story Two: Maggie Masters Mayhem

Maggie had been home all day with her three kids and had just plain had enough. Her three-year-old had "fixed" the carpet stains with magic marker, her five-year-old had "cooked" with every pot and pan in the kitchen, and the seven-year-old had "done" his homework by tying a pen onto the dog's tail (in hopes that the dog would "write" the answers on the worksheets). She had pleaded and bribed for quiet to no avail, before she remembered the sermon she had heard in church the prior Sunday.

The pastor had suggested that each person could call on spiritual forces to command change. *Why not?* Maggie thought. *Nothing else has worked!* The idea of calling on the spirit or force of calm entered her mind. Taking a deep breath, Maggie summoned this force and said, "Quiet!"

The children stopped moving. Maggie marveled. Staying connected to this supernatural force, she gave instructions for picking up that were actually obeyed. When she finally began cooking dinner, she peeped out to see whether "the force" was still working. The children were sleeping in front of the television.

Story Three: Assiz Hopes for Happiness

Assiz had seen so many doctors and therapists that he felt like giving up on himself, which was actually his problem! He had been depressed for many years. Nothing seemed to offer cheer; no advice or pill worked. He didn't know what to do.

In despair, he decided he needed to do think outside the box. Taking a day off work, he sat down by a nearby river. In a book, he had read that healers and people with special gifts used to do something called divining, which involved looking into a mirror or water for a sign. As he peered into the water, he hoped to see an omen, an image, or anything that could indicate the key to happiness. A picture did materialize in the water, but at first he discounted it. His own face reflected back to him. The longer he gazed at the image, however, the more applicable the image became.

The Assiz in the water appeared happy, not sad. His eyes were calm and wise, not distraught and dismayed. Assiz felt as if the mirror image might smile or laugh at any moment! In a flash of inspiration, Assiz decided to "switch places" with this magic self, to release the depressed Assiz in the river in exchange for the happy Assiz.

Assiz felt odd the rest of the day, like he was buzzing or tingling. He went to bed with a slight headache, but he woke up feeling fine. In fact, he felt more than fine—he felt great! As the week progressed, he continued to feel better and better, as if he had transformed into a "being of light" rather than a "shadow of the dark." His inner personality continued to evolve until, months later, he felt that he was cured of depression.

Story Four: The Priest Prays for Healing

Noreen could hardly lift her hand. "Thanks for coming to visit me," she said to her parish priest, Father Bryan. Noreen had been diagnosed with terminal cancer. In an act of faith and desperation, her mother had asked the parish priest to visit and pray for Noreen's health.

Father Bryan was a soft-spoken, humble man. It was rumored that his prayers had effected healing in a child in his last parish. Noreen's mother had uncovered this story and pleaded for a personal visit.

Father Bryan didn't like the pressure, but agreed to visit, stating that the healing was in God's hands, not his own. With hope in his heart and a prayer on his lips, he asked God to heal Noreen. She slipped into a quiet sleep and the priest left.

Noreen woke from her sleep feeling refreshed for the first time in months. As the day progressed, she felt better and better. A test a week later confirmed what she perceived was occurring in her body. The cancer was gone. Noreen and her parents attributed the miracle to Father Bryan's prayers; he gave praise to God.

Have you found yourself in similar experiences?

We start with what we call "reality" in Story One, which reveals common sense and commonplace as the norm. We've all been guilty of magical thinking, when we simply ought to sit down and do some practical thinking! Joseph's dilapidated car wasn't jinxed by jinn or zapped by the supernatural. It was old and falling apart. The *elemental pathway*, as depicted in this story, is the normal, the everyday, the predictable—and that has its own special brand of magic.

Story Two depicts the *power pathway*. This pathway supervises the supernatural, the land of forces and energies that, if directed, result in extraordinary outcomes. Have you ever concentrated so hard that an influence more powerful than you can explain "takes over"? Then you have employed the strength of the power pathway, the contact point to the paranormal.

Review Story Three and you enter the *imagination pathway*, the world of creative magic. Assiz was pushed to his emotional limit, right up against the boundaries between this world and the antiworld, the place of possibilities available to us all. Through your imagination, you exchange this reality for a better one, using a form of magic available to everyone.

Story Four shows how heaven weaves through earth, sometimes erasing what shouldn't be. Noreen experienced the miracles of the *divine pathway* as Father Bryan prayed for healing. Here, we open our hearts to the love of the Divine.

You are already an expert at each pathway. You have plotted the particulars of the elemental pathway and surfed the supernatural energies of the power pathway. You have created with the mystery of the imagination pathway and secured the sacred on the divine pathway. You ARE elemental, empowered, imaginative, and divine.

Perhaps the best image for describing your relationship with the pathways and the Greater Reality is to picture a chessboard made of four stacked layers. Each of these levels is a pathway. Now draw multiple lines between each layer so the final figure resembles a multiconnected swirl.

If you keep observing, you'll notice that this multidimensional figure interconnects with other figures, objects, beings, and places. The sum total is the Greater Reality, which is made of light.

Ultimately, our hearts heal once we fully understand that we are really made of light, a light that is always nourished by the Greater Light. How do we work with these threads or pathways of light? By understanding them.

1. The Elemental Pathway: Physical Reality

The word *elemental* means fundamental. Working with the elemental pathway involves a process called *reduction*, the act of breaking down a situation into its component parts. When seeking to heal a heart condition, you begin by analyzing the problem and its causes. Your healing methods depend upon the causes of the heart condition.

Most healing modalities are based on elemental healing, including Western and Eastern medicine, traditional and holistic health care, and emotional and mental therapeutic processes. Through the perspective of the Four Pathways approach, you can generate great change with small actions. Let's say you begin eating a heart-healthy diet, an obvious elemental strategy for heart healing. By also focusing on one or all of the other pathways, you engineer healing on other pathways, thus calling healing energies from these pathways into your process. You could combine a power force with your food and supercharge your nutrients; imagine magical properties into your food and invite a miracle; or ask the Divine to bless your food and receive peace and calm while eating. How can an act as simple as eating a healthy meal produce such substantial change? Remember that even when working with the elemental pathway, which seems the most familiar because it operates within our physical world, you are working with informed vibration.

To achieve phenomenal elemental pathway results, employ the tool of *intention*. When you intend a result at the level of 110 percent, you will get it! All the pathways will shift to support your goal.

2. The Power Pathway: Supernatural Strength

On the power pathway, heart disease is healed through the direct manipulation of supernatural energies and forces. Through the power pathway, you can spin away the energy creating heart problems or add energies that can strengthen your body's healing abilities.

Most healers, especially shamans and medicine workers, understand that the invisible world is as real as the visible. To excel at the power pathway, you must learn how to read and summon the forces underneath physical reality. An example of power pathway healing for heart disease includes checking for supernatural forces and energies that create distortions about love and upset the natural balance of the heart's processes. Upon identifying these distorting influences, a power player would use positive forces to create change.

Change occurs on the power pathway through *commanding*. You cannot command change unless you claim your right to be a cocreator of the physical universe, starting with your own body. Chapter 7, Shift Healing on the Power Pathway, can teach you the basics regarding available forces and powers, but only you can assert the authority needed to use this pathway calmly and ethically.

3. The Imagination Pathway: Creative Magic

Your imagination is your finest healing tool, more precise and incisive than a surgical instrument. Scientifically, the imagination pathway is the space that links this world and the antiworld. If you have heart disease, your heart issues exist in this world. There is also a "you" that doesn't have heart disease. That self lingers in one of the many antiworlds, or parallel universes, accessible to you through your imagination.

Why is this pathway deemed *creative magic*? Think of what might happen if you could, through the door of the imagination, exchange your unhealthy heart for a healed one. The result is

magical! By applying the healing tool of *imagining*, you can transform possibilities into realities.

4. The Divine Pathway: Awakening to Love

The divine pathway is synonymous with heart healing, as it
is fundamentally about love. On the divine pathway, a heart
disorder represents an attempt, however misguided, to give,
receive, or learn about love. Through the lens of the divine pathway, the unhealthy heart is actually perceived as a healthy heart;
it is questing for love and that is what counts.

Many of us are unwilling to be transparent enough to allow
divine healing. We don't like being vulnerable. If we're to receive
the blessings available on the divine pathway, we must decide to
be vulnerable. *Petitioning* begins the process of divine healing, as
it forces us to open our hearts to the Divine. Petitioning isn't a
religious act, nor does it necessarily involve traditional prayer or
meditation. To petition is to share your deepest need and profess
a willingness to be loved.

On the divine pathway, whatever or whoever is available to
deliver the healing will respond. You might ask for a good surgeon, and the divine pathway will drop a magazine article into
your lap. Then again, you might request a surgeon and a neighbor
drops by to pray with you, or an angel does the favor in your
dreams. Be assured that the Divine will heal you according to
divine will. If this pathway results in miracles, it is because the
Divine ultimately dictates the laws of science, not the other way
around.

Chakras on the Four Pathways

All four pathways flow into the Greater Reality, even as each
functions independently. Imagine our three-dimensional
chessboard again, the one with all the lines and connections.
How do you traverse from one level to another? How do you deal

with the infinite variations of healing? You do so through your chakras, energy organs that serve as portals between the pathways.

Most metaphysicians, including myself, see chakras with the inner eye as swirling and conical-shaped vortexes. There are subtle energy threads between each chakra and another set of energy organs called the auric field. Twelve basic chakras, centers that regulate the "you inside of you," match with twelve fundamental auric bands, wave bands that manage the "you outside of you." Both of these sets of energies serve a vital purpose in shift healing.

To perform Four Pathways healing, you will work with twelve basic chakras. Seven chakras are located directly in your physical body and five are outside of the body proper. Although there are many chakras in the human energy system (the total network of energy organs that regulate your existence), these twelve enable diagnosis and healing.

All chakras share several commonalities. Each regulates a specific set of physical, mental, emotional, and spiritual concerns. They are somewhat uniform in shape, appearing as swirling vortexes that move in tighter circles when closer to the body and bigger circles when farther away. They all are energetic organs. This means that they operate on frequencies or vibrations and are able to process all types or speeds of energy. As energy organs, they can convert tachyon (fast-moving energies) into quark (slow-moving energies). The result is phenomenal! Through your chakras, you can make energies appear or disappear. Conceivably, you could wink a diseased artery out of your body and snap in a healthy one. By deliberately programming your chakras for health, you can attract universal energies to support your well-being.

I stress again that chakras are also physical organs. Each is based in at least one endocrine gland or hormone-producing organ and operates a certain section of the material body. This is why it is advantageous to work with chakras: What you do emotionally, mentally, spiritually, or psychically can impact your physical health.

Chakras also differ from each other. Each vibrates on a different speed and processes a unique set of information. The heart chakra, for instance, a major concern in heart disease, manages the organs of your chest, emotions connected to relationship, beliefs about love, and your spiritual connection with the Divine. Yet another chakra, the first chakra, works with your adrenals, feelings about yourself, beliefs about security, and the spirituality of a personal identity.

When seeking to heal heart disease, you might assume that you will always work with the heart chakra. Typically, the heart chakra is involved in a heart condition, but the heart chakra may not be your focus chakra. Heart disease isn't always rooted in the heart. Consider diabetes. People often develop heart problems in the later stages of diabetes, an illness that originates in the pancreas, an organ located in the third chakra. If you have diabetes-related heart disease, on the Four Pathways system you will perform considerable work in the third chakra. In this approach, you will always select a *primary disease chakra*, the chakra that oversees the processes creating disruption in the heart. You might also work with a *secondary disease chakra*, the chakra that is home to the secondary cause of the disease.

Why work with a chakra instead of a physical organ or body site? Think of how much more effective and faster your healing process will be if you work energetically in addition to physically. By working with a chakra, you can perform functions greatly expanded beyond those provided by the major medical model. For instance, you can do the following:

1. Determine which pathway(s) holds the origin of your heart condition. It's always best to heal at the source.
2. Pinpoint the chakra, and therefore bodily organs, causing your heart trouble. Heart disease doesn't always stem from problems in the heart muscle or vessels. Again, it's more effective to heal a disease at the source.

3. Diagnose for the true causes of the heart condition. By working with the chakras, you can review hundreds of physical, emotional, mental, spiritual, and potential causes, greatly expanding beyond the medical toolbox.

4. Shift or transfer healing energies from one pathway to another and ultimately into the chakra that can best repair your body. Chakras can act as transformers, adapting energies that can be too strong or powerful for your physical body, thus gently providing healing and support.

You will perform chakra magic with your psychic abilities. We all have innate psychic gifts. When employed consciously and conscientiously, these inherent but often uncontrolled capabilities transform into intuitive skills. You can focus your specific intuitive skills to gain perceptions, information, and interpretations of informed vibration, and also to shape, change, and move energies for healing. In chapter 5, you will take a quiz that will help you pinpoint your particular intuitive style.

Knowledge about your gifts can help you accomplish two major goals: energy mapping for a disease's causes and healing ideas, and shift healing to accomplish change. Energy mapping involves creating pictorial representations of the causes of a heart problem. An energy map is key to deciding how to conduct shift healing.

Pathway healing will frequently necessitate working with your auric bands as well as your chakras. These bands look and function a little differently on each pathway; nonetheless, they always serve some basic tasks: to provide protection and boundaries and to attract energies needed for health and happiness. By working with the paired set of a chakra and an auric band, you can engineer healing inside of the body and lock it in outside of the body. You can alter an errant pattern in your heart and attract only the energies that will support the change you want. You can heal inside and out.

There are dozens of other energy bodies that can be tapped into for health and healing. You'll be introduced to many of them in Part II of this book, where I explore the specific contours of each pathway. Vital to pathway healing is grasping the underlying principle that all healing involves working energetically. In the next chapter, we'll take a look at the specifics of energetic healing as it pertains to heart disease. I'll show you why you can benefit from pathway healing, and the real meaning, from an energetic perspective, of heart disease. You may be surprised by this new way of looking at yourself.

The Energy of Heart Disease

The supreme heaven shines in the lotus of the heart. They enter there who struggle and aspire.

—*Kaivalya Upanishad*†

I f we exist in the Greater Reality, in heaven on earth, then we must ask what causes the development of heart disease. If in the Greater Reality all is love, and love and heart problems can't coexist, then what creates the conditions of lack of love in our hearts and in our lives? It's easiest to answer this question by considering an energetic interpretation of heart disease.

Our Hurting Hearts

Statistically, many of us either already have or will develop what we call a "bad heart." Our fear about heart trouble is one reason that the heart is the organ most frequently discussed, analyzed, researched, and written about in the scientific community. Consider these statistics from the United States in 2005: [1]

- An American life is lost to heart attack every 33 seconds. More than 1.5 million Americans have heart attacks each

†*The Upanishads—Breath of the Eternal, trans.* Swami Prabhavananda and Frederick Manchester (New York: Signet Classics, 2002), p. 114.

year, and, of these, more than 300,000 people who suffer an attack die before reaching a hospital.

- For one-third of these people, the attack was the first sign of a heart problem.
- One out of every two deaths in the United States is due to heart disease or stroke. An astonishing 42 percent of women die within the year following a heart attack, compared to 24 percent of men.
- Hypertension, one type of heart disease, affects more than 63 million Americans, yet 35 percent of people with hypertension do not know they have the condition.
- About one-sixth of people who die of heart troubles are under age sixty-five.
- More than half of all Americans have cholesterol levels higher than 200 mg/dL, the point at which the risk for heart troubles rises. After age fifty, women's counts are higher than men's.
- Stroke, a product of heart problems, is the third leading cause of death in the United States. It is also the leading origin of disability. Sixty-one percent or more of stroke victims are women.

It is commonly known that factors such as genetics, obesity, hypertension, and smoking create conditions for heart disease, but it's becoming evident that there is more to the heart than its physicality. Scientists agree that emotional states, including stress, anxiety, hostility, and depression, are just as likely to cause heart illness as anything physical. And, as pointed out by Edward Suarez, associate professor of psychiatry and human behavior at Duke University, "Fifty percent of people who have heart attacks do not have high cholesterol."[2]

Consider as well research proving an association among stress, emotions, and cardiovascular disease. In a study at Duke University, hostile people, as measured by a standardized test, displayed a 29 percent greater chance of dying of heart disease, and this figure jumped to more than 50 percent in people sixty and older.[3] All stresses, including childhood trauma, can create the conditions for heart disease. In a survey of 17,000 adults in San Diego, Dr. Maxia Dong at the Centers for Disease Control and Prevention found that the risk of a heart attack was 30 to 70 percent higher in people who had suffered adverse childhood experiences, such as abuse, family alcoholism, or domestic violence.[4]

What characterizes our current sociological environment is the inordinate amount of fear—a severe emptiness indicating lack of self-love—that causes people to turn to workaholism, addictions, abusive behavior, codependency, and self-hatred. As a whole, we must pay attention to the voices in our hearts, the heart of our hearts, if we are to heal ourselves.

The Heart of the Heart

The heart has always been seen as something more than a physical organ. Spiritually, the heart has been elevated as the seat of great wisdom and love. The ancient Egyptians measured the worth of a person by his or her heart. At death, proclaimed the Egyptians, the goddess of justice would weigh the deceased person's heart against the weight of a feather. A "light heart" was free from transgression.

The same idea holds true in many religions. In Hinduism, the heart is referenced as the seat of Atman, the human equivalent of the Absolute, or Brahman. In Islam, the heart is the temporal house of the spirit and knowing. And in Christianity, the heart is believed to house an essence not visible to the naked eye, though this essence is ultimately the measure of our relationship with the Creator. As stated in I Samuel 16:7, man "looketh on the outward appearance, but the Lord looketh on the heart."

Consider the notion of the heart as the seat of romantic love, popularized in the Middle Ages onward. Thanks to the romanticists, we now send valentines frilly with lace every February 14.

This puffy interpretation of the heart was counterbalanced by other religious images, especially those of the Christian variety, in which the hearts of the various saints, Mother Mary, and Jesus were depicted as suffering for the sins of the people. Even now, postcards of Jesus or Mary from the Vatican are often depicted with larger-than-life hearts or arrows piercing their hearts.

These illustrations all present the heart as basically good and decent, but there are also thoughts contrary to that idea. In Matthew 15:18–19, Jesus points out that the heart can house hate as well as love, in observing that "what comes out of the mouth proceeds from the heart, and this defiles a man. For out of the heart come evil thoughts, murder, adultery, fornication, theft, false witness, slander."

His Holiness the Dalai Lama, the spiritual leader of the New Kadam School of Tibetan Buddhism, affirms a Buddhist view similar to that of Christianity. In the end, following the Buddhist discipline is an attainment of *dharmakaya*, the Truth Body of the Buddha. *Dharmakaya* refers to seeing the Buddha, a by-product of pursuing the light of wisdom and knowledge, while turning away from the darkness of ignorance and lack of knowledge.[5]

Light and dark exist simultaneously in the heart. When you make the hard choice to choose only light, you are on the path to enlightenment. There are many terms for the state of enlightenment, including being born again, illuminated, spiritual, and ascended. In the Four Pathways system, I use the term *wakefulness* to avoid the dualistic association of dark with evil and light with good.

Gary Zukav connects quantum physics with the pursuit of enlightenment in his book, *The Seat of the Soul*. Shares Zukav, "You are a system of Light, as are all beings. The frequency of your Light depends upon your consciousness. When you shift your consciousness, you shift the frequency of your Light."[6] Zukav then offers suggestions for making these shifts, all of which are based on variations of love, such as employing affection, joy, and compassion.

In dealing with heart disease, the most important chakra to engage is most likely the heart chakra, which enfolds the heart, lungs, breasts, and chest area, front and back. Dr. Richard Gerber, a pioneer in vibrational medicine, emphasizes both the spiritual and the physical nature of the heart chakra in his groundbreaking book, *Vibrational Medicine*. Shares Dr. Gerber, "The reason that the heart center is so significant is that an open heart is integral to an individual's ability to express love." Unless we develop our inner heart, Gerber states, we'll continue to see a "tremendous mortality due to heart disease."[7]

Gerber relates the Western world's extreme incidence of coronary artery disease, heart attacks, and other circulatory diseases, such as stroke, to the following factors:[8]

- Reduction of energy through the heart chakra causes stagnation of blood flow.
- Stasis of energy flow through the heart chambers can result in formation of blood clots.
- Beliefs and expressions of love impact the respiratory system, which interacts crucially with the physical heart.

Gerber wasn't the first to make the leap from the heart to a person's physical well-being. Among the ancient Maya, the human being was seen as a pyramidal energy structure. The Maya believed that breathing activates bioelectromagnetic energy that stimulates physical cells and the heart, which then "conveys bioelectric current to the muscles, organs and bodily systems and keeps them alive."[9]

The twelfth-century Persian Sufis also linked the heart with physical health as well as higher truths. The Sufis believed the heart chakra not only regulates the circulatory system but also establishes the parameters for the entirety of life. In fact, the Sufis followed a spiritual belief system often called "the way of the heart." They asserted that reality was organized in several *hadarats*, or planes of reality. These levels of reality synchronize with the four pathways.[10]

Essentially, healing the heart always boils down to working with love. In the Four Pathways model, love isn't simply an idea or a concept. It is the end goal of the journey of the pathways, culminating in the Greater Reality.

The Energetics of Love

Love is the most powerful energy in the world. It can alter a person, a relationship, a family, a community, or the world. Love can also change the physical nature of the heart because, in its various forms, it can produce tangible results.

Love is a form of energy that can be tracked, applied, and directed for greater healing.

There are many types of love, including compassion, empathy, understanding, acceptance, appreciation, and gratitude. All shapes and sizes of love produce a measurable and positive effect on the body in general and the heart in particular, and this can now be measured scientifically and validated through theories based on physics.

One interesting set of studies reveals the physiological benefits of appreciation, as defined as a sense of wonder that can be directed toward yourself or another.[11] In one study, participants who consciously felt the feeling of appreciation and love not only enjoyed smooth and healthy heart rhythms but also a synchronization among other bodily systems, which in turn promoted efficiency, regeneration, higher cognition, emotional stability, and an overall greater quality of life.[12]

Empathy is yet another form of love. When empathy is present between people, it results in physical changes in the heart, as shown in a study conducted by professors Levenson and Gottman at the University of California at Berkeley. Research revealed that physiological changes occurred between married couples during empathetic interactions. The best results were noted between couples that showed they cared about each other's needs, as determined by verbal interactions on various subjects. The physiological markers of these highly empathetic couples mimicked each other while empathizing. If one partner's heart rate went up, so did the others; if one went down, so did the others. This and other studies have led to the term *cardioelectromagnetic communication*, used by heart-energy expert Dr. Rollin McCraty to explain how the nervous system acts like an antenna that responds to the connection between individual's magnetic heart fields.[13] Hence, proof of what we intrinsically know: The heart is about love and love controls the body.

Some of the effects of love can be explained through a concept called "coherence." *Coherence* refers to the distribution of power in a wave. The more stable the frequency and shape of a waveform, the higher coherence—and the better the functionality and health—of the organ emanating that wave. For example, a coherent heartbeat is orderly and stable. A coherent heart pumps blood methodically and easily, reducing your risk of heart attack, stroke, or other problems.

Auto-coherency means that an organ's waveforms are internally stable. A heart with auto-coherency will tend toward health as long as it vibrates according to its correct *resonance*, or natural frequency. Auto-coherence, however, isn't enough to provide health. Your heart also needs to have resonance with other organs or physical systems, because everything in the body is interdependent.

Cross-coherency is the term used to show the relationship between or among different systems. When your heart's patterns are stable, they enter into a cross-coherent relationship called *entrainment* with other organs or physical systems. Entrained frequencies affect each other and can eventually arrive at the same vibration or harmony. When this entrainment supports the resonance of each organ's frequency, you have optimum health. An example of a positive cross-coherent relationship is that which exists between your circulatory and respiratory systems. You can calm your heart with deep breaths, and a calm heart will enhance the health of your respiratory system.

The heart entrains to many other organs and systems, which is why it is an ideal organ for delivering love and its healing effects throughout the body. In *The Appreciative Heart*, author Dr. Rollin McCraty shows how changes in the heart produce changes throughout the body, such as in the respiratory, digestive, and neurological systems, and in the brain and skin.[14] If you consider the fact that entrainment can occur between any oscillating or vibrating unit, then we must recognize that the heart can entrain to EVERYTHING in the body. ANY loving emotion, feeling, or spiritual truth, when focused through the heart, increases the coherency of the heart and positively affects all systems. Concentrate on negative emotions, such as anger, frustration, or anxiety, and the opposite happens. The heart becomes physically less coherent—and therefore less healthy—as do other parts of the body.[15] Love can help make you healthy, while lack of love can make you sick.

In the Greater Reality, there is only love. Love enhances. It allows. It invites. It heals. The reason there is disease, trauma, abuse, and suffering is that most of us organize our lives around something that is not love. What is this something? We must understand the "enemy" if we are to better help our hearts.

Fear and the Heart

Many spiritual practices, philosophers, and writers suggest that fear is the opposite of love, therefore the root of all the world's problems. I agree with this, but I also define fear differently than most people do. Whereas fear is usually thought of as a "something"—an energy, a feeling, a belief, or a set of chemical reactions—I see fear as absolutely nothing.

> FEAR ISN'T THE PRESENCE OF ANYTHING; IT IS THE ABSENCE OF LOVE. IF we're not loved thoroughly when growing up, we form our perceptions, ideas, and feelings around an internal emptiness, the space that should have been filled with love. We then live the rest of our lives simultaneously seeking to fill this space while trying not to be swallowed up by it.

How can we be frightened of the love that would fill the emptiness? Why would we refuse the cure for our heart problems? Imagine that you are standing in the empty space within your own heart. Attempt to feel the love that the Divine, the world, and your loved ones have been holding for you. Our entire lives are based on attempts to get love, but if we're really honest with ourselves, we will see that we have never really acted in such a way as to be open to "real" love. There are lots of artificial forms of love, including sex, drugs, food, work, busyness, socializing, and addictive behaviors and substances. But if we were to actually internalize real love, the following would have to occur:

1. We would have to acknowledge the fact that love has been missing, and this is a painful admission.

2. We would feel the pain of having missed out on love.

3. We would review our own behavior and find ourselves lacking. People void of love seldom give "real love" to others. They are either codependent, giving in order to get back, or closed-hearted, refusing any exchange.

4. We would have to feel the shame that crawls into all empty spaces. Shame tells us that we weren't loved because we were "bad."

5. We would have to be brave enough to determine whether the shame-based messages are true or not.

Let me provide an example.

Marcus was a well-known president of a multinational company. At age forty-five, he had already experienced two heart attacks. He came to see me because he wanted to learn how to meditate.

Meditation is a fine way to calm a disgruntled heart, but it won't settle really turbulent emotional waters. To help Marcus, we needed to find out why he hated himself enough to attack his own heart.

I used regression methods on the elemental pathway to travel back in time, asking to unearth the inner self who had perceived himself as unloved. Marcus returned to being four years of age. At the time, his father was working all the time. When he was present, he treated Marcus with disdain and cruelty. The only trait Marcus admired in his father was his financial success. Lacking his father's attention and approval, Marcus decided that when he grew up he would become even more successful than his father. Then his father would love him! Marcus sealed the empty space, the place where he needed his father's love, with the belief that his father didn't love him because there was something wrong with him. He would allow himself to be loved only when he was successful enough to earn it.

Marcus had spent the better part of forty years "earning his father's love." He worked nonstop, bringing each success to his father like a cat delivers a bird to its master's doorstep. Did he ever really succeed? Did his dad ever say, "Good job, I'm proud of you"? His dad was more likely to sniff and change the subject than he was to bestow a compliment. Marcus tried harder, all the time avoiding the empty spot that lay in the center of his life, in the center of his heart.

During our sessions, Marcus resisted dealing with his feelings about his father. He even walked out one day, saying he was tired of wasting his time. I knew why. Marcus was afraid the emptiness reflected the truth about him. Maybe he didn't deserve love. Maybe he was unlovable, unworthy of even the slightest shred of compassion. Then one day, everything changed for Marcus. He broke down and began to cry. All he had ever wanted was to be loved, and he wasn't ever going to fill this need with anything his father could provide.

As he delved into this sad truth, Marcus began to see that once he did have love in his life, but he had turned it away because of shame and emptiness. His wife had just left him; he didn't even remember his daughters' birthdays. Marcus was a working machine, a man who had forgotten where he had left his heart, which was in the emptiness within his heart. In "attacking his father" for love, Marcus had only succeeded in attacking himself.

As his therapy progressed, Marcus stopped holding out for love. He developed new ways of seeing himself that led toward more loving behavior, such as better dietary and exercise habits. He started calling his daughters on the phone, and eventually spent more time with them. He drifted away from our sessions as he became happier in his life. Five years after he began working with me, he called. His doctors had pronounced his heart "healthy."

As with my work with Marcus, I almost always perceive an empty space centered in the heart of someone with heart disease. Sometimes this space is partially filled with other energies, such as negative or self-alienating beliefs or shame and fear-based feelings. Sometimes a modicum of love has crept in, just enough to pose the question, "Do I deserve more love?" The job is to finish filling this space called "fear" with love.

The Opportunity of Heart Disease

You can't necessarily return for love to the person or situation that originally created your lovelessness. You might not be able to count on your current companions for the love that you need. The voice of love, however, is always present. It lies within your heart, which is whole within the Greater Reality. Love might only be one voice among many, but it is always the true voice among the millions of dissidents.

If you have heart disease, you have been entrusted with the opportunity to enter the emptiness of the past and open yourself to the love that awaits. Love is always present, even if you can't see it in your life at this time. Love is your birthright. It is the path through life. The Divine clapped in glee when you were conceived and cushioned you through the birth canal. The Divine welcomed you into the world and offered wisdom and handkerchiefs when you sorrowed. And the Divine stands ready to embrace you when it's time to leave, inviting you back into God's heart.

If you don't feel loved, it might be that you don't know how to perceive yourself as loved. Science has proven that an observer affects the outcome of an experiment. Perhaps you must stop looking at yourself with your current eyes and instead see yourself through the eyes of God. That act would create you as both the observer and the observed—and show you that you are loved.

The Boulevard of Energy

You are standing at a crossroads, staring at a map trying to decide how to proceed. There are two obvious roads forward. The Avenue of Logic is dark and murky, but it is well traveled. Select this road and you reiterate the fear that causes heart problems, but you won't feel alone, for there are countless aids along the way. There are clinics with tried-and-true techniques, and statistics that suggest you have "a chance." Of course, you could strike out on the Street of Hope, but this choice seems so . . . illogical. Certainly, the Street of Hope is brightly and even gaily lit, but there are so few others on this course. The map outlines virtues like faith and truth in contrast to the clinical buildings sketched on the Avenue of Logic, and there's not a statistic to be seen, merely ideas like "promises of the Divine" and "the healing power of Love." How can anyone guarantee the efficacy of hope? This choice seems so unfair!

And it is. You look closer, hoping to spy an alternative. If you strain really hard, you notice that there is one. Can you make out the words? Energy Boulevard, the Key to the Four Pathways System. What's this, you wonder? As you peer closer, it's as if the figures, buildings, words, and assurances outlined along the boulevard spring to life. Logic and love combine to create healing and health; prayers mix with potions, and medicines make a difference. On the Energy Boulevard, you don't have to choose between logic and hope, reason and love; the Four Pathways system affords all realities because it works through the reality of energy.

By understanding energy, you engage the practical and the possible, and create the reality of healing.

How Energy Works

Working energetically is the most effective way to allow heart healing, no matter the pathway, because all illnesses reduce to energetic imbalances. We only have to work with the basics of reality to shift reality.

I've discussed two of the many types of quanta that compose reality. There are the quarks, our relatively slow-moving friends, who prefer "snail mail" to the zip-speed of tachyons, our faster-than-light message deliverers. We can convert a quark to a tachyon and back again; in fact, we can alter just about any energy from particle to waveform and vice versa. Once we are able to do this, we are versatile enough to maneuver time, space, and anything in between.

Science used to believe that matter was trapped in time and space, that a rock could only be destroyed by force or erosion. Now research in quantum physics suggests that at any point you could blink the rock right out of existence—say, to the moment before it was formed—or you could transform it into a mountain! This means that at any point in time, you can also shift away heart disease using quantum physics. Recent experiments reveal that "quantum fields are not mediated by forces but by exchange of energy, which is constantly redistributed in a dynamic pattern."[16] Since everything that exists is a field, you can alter the attitude, gene, pattern, issue, historical fact, or emotion that is underlying the disease and exchange it for a healthier thought, consciousness, habit, chromosome, memory, or feeling.

Research conducted by Dr. Emoto of Japan reveals the phenomenal power of conscious energy shifting. Using prayer, music, or written intentions, Dr. Emoto has altered the crystalline structure of water molecules. Positive, spiritually based messages produce beautiful molecular patterns, while hateful messages result in gloomy, ugly patterns.[17]

Sometimes the most phenomenal results occur when two people interface. In one study, scientists used an electroencephalogram (EEG) to see what happened when two people touched. One person's electrocardiograph signal registered on the other person's in the heart and also elsewhere on the body.[18] We affect each other. Made of energy, we can share, trade, and heal each other energetically. This includes altering the energy of heart disease.

The Vibration of Heart Disease

Changing your energetic program from fear to love will alter the vibration of your heart and create healing. You can also modify the vibration to encourage love and thus promote a healthy heart. You don't have to be a physics professor to work with vibration on the Four Pathways system, but it is helpful to grasp the basic concepts.

Our daily lives do not require most of us to distinguish between movement and vibration, but the two are in fact different. Movement indicates a shift from one space to another, whereas vibration is movement that involves a change of direction. When something vibrates it not only moves from one space to another, it also moves up or down, back and forth, or in circles. Healing is all about consciously deciding the direction in which something should vibrate instead of letting your subconscious decide.

Many forms of energy vibrate in measurable and consistent ways. Sound waves are one form of predictable, vibrating energy, as are radio waves, light, and any other type of oscillating energy. A vibrating object's rate of intensity can be determined by the information encoded within it. Change the vibration and you change the information.

We usually think that vibration is orderly, but it's not. Most particles oscillate in several, if not hundreds, of directions, sometimes hitting the corners of other worlds as well! Your heart, for instance, has an overall vibration, but each part and particle of the heart has its own vibration.

The overall or observable vibration of a moving particle, wave, or other unit of energy is called a *frequency*. Your heart is attuned to an optimum frequency, as are all other parts of you. If an organ is playing out of tune with the rest of the body, we call the result a disease, or a "lack of ease," within the system.

Your heart's erratic frequency isn't necessarily caused by a bad program or vibration in the heart. Of the twelve major chakras, eleven have direct influence on the heart. The twelfth chakra connects to the body at thirty-two different contact points and is therefore indirectly, rather than directly, related to heart health. If another physical organ is highly discordant, it can eventually cause disharmony in the heart. Because of cross-coherence, problems anywhere in the body, mind, or soul can cause heart troubles. For instance, fatty food can upset the liver, a major gland located in the third chakra. In response, the liver might churn out too much cholesterol, which builds up as plaque in the circulatory system, eventually creating the conditions for a heart attack.

Of major importance in pathway healing is to determine your personal *harmonic*, a set of tones that emanate from your spirit, or Greater Self. All parts of you operate on different frequencies—as does everything in the universe. What makes your spirit unique is that its tones are all created from spiritual truths like faith, hope, truth, and love. From a physic's point of view, these spiritual truths form *standing waveforms*, shafts of energy that connect seemingly opposing energies. For instance, your spirit is able to link a truth like love with the imperfect feeling of fear, and then convert your fears into opportunities to love.

Your spirit's methods for doing this type of creative healing and manifesting are personal. The end result, if you could hear your spirit perform this function, would be a medley or concerto that serves as your own personality blueprint. This concluding song is your own spiritual harmonic.

If you attune to your spiritual harmonic in all you do, your body will be healthy. The spiritual truths inherent in your Greater Self will not only cancel out the harmful effects of any dysfunctional genes, behaviors, or ideas but will actually transform them into positives—thus the healing action of the Greater Self's ability to create standing wave forms. If you deliberately live from your harmonic, your body can cope with and find uses for all your problems. Any part of you in discord with the core harmonic is vulnerable to disease. Heart disease indicates a separation between your spirit's basic harmonic about love and the love frequencies held in your body; it is a lack of resonance.

Disease involves both inaccurate information and destructive vibrations. Your heart, more than any other organ, is particularly sensitive to "bad vibrations" because it is the center of your electromagnetic system. The heart processes energy from the lower, more physical chakras as well as the higher, more spiritual chakras, and thus is responsible for exchanging information about the earth with information from the heavens.

Other Energy Factors in Healing

There are several other factors to consider when working with the pathways to heal heart disease with quantum-based energy theory.

Time and Space I like to work interdimensionally when seeking to heal heart disease. To do so, it's helpful to understand the basics of current spacetime theory.

Although scientists theorize that there are ten dimensions interconnected by "strings," I work with thirteen. String theory postulates that the fundamental units that make up what we perceive as reality are in fact miniscule strands of energy that are one trillionth of one trillionth the size of an atom. These strands, also called strings, have small tails, or whips, that vibrate. Some strings might connect to many dimensions at the same time, while others stay in one dimension primarily.

Like all matter, we are composed of umpteen strings. Because strings are interconnected within different dimensions, we are interconnected—and exist upon—all dimensions simultaneously. This means that the cause of heart disease could actually lie in different dimensions. It also means that you could shift energies from other dimensions to heal heart disease.

Current heart theory from the Institute of HeartMath suggests that information is encoded or recorded during the intervals between nerve impulses, hormone pulses, or the pressures of blood and electromagnetic waves produced by the heart.[19] Seeing time as malleable—as nonexistent between beats or pulses—ironically gives you plenty of time to reprogram your heart for healing. As meditation experts, gurus, and healers across the ages have done, you can learn how to control your consciousness, enter the space between your heartbeats, and unlock the love inside. Working within various pathways, you can encode your heart, or any other causative organ, with the symbols, energies, healing powers, or even memories necessary for a turnaround in health.

Using this technique, you can alter the past, present, or future. Think of how many opportunities your heart provides you for these healing moments. *The average heart beats about 2.5 billion times during a lifetime. That's a lot of spaces between beats in which to perform healing!*

Fields and Forces Most pathway healing involves working with fields and forces. We know that everything vibrates, which means that everything is in motion. Motion creates a field around all objects, animate or not. *Fields* are energetic extensions or waves that emanate from their source. Some fields create *forces*, such as electrical, weak or strong nuclear, magnetic, or electromagnetic forces. The information telling a field or force what to do and how to do it can either cause or cure heart disease. Conversely, the vibration of and information held within a field can either cause or cure heart disease.

Long ago, a researcher named Harold Saxton Burr was convinced that fields actually instruct the body rather than the other way around. He was able to detect cancer in people's fields before they were diagnosed, showing that what we pick up energetically can affect our physical health.[20] We can use this same capability to diagnose heart disease, either through the auric band related to the primary disease chakra or through the heart field itself.

We exist within several electromagnetic and other energy fields, not only those generated from inside our body. While the heart is certainly affected by vibrations within its own structure, it is also altered by energies outside of itself and the body temporal. Dr. Richard Gerber discusses several studies that underscore this point in his book *A Practical Guide to Vibrational Medicine*. French research shows a strong connection between heart attack incidents and strong solar-flare activity, when a small area of the sun's surface temporarily emits bursts of energy. Solar-energy bursts cause alterations in the earth's magnetic field, which might explain the correlation between the intensity of the solar flare and the rate of reported heart trouble. The heart is an electromagnetic organ, and intense changes in the magnetic fields surrounding the body can shock the heart. Other geobiologists have confirmed this association, revealing a correspondence among blood clotting, the entire cardiovascular system, and sunspots, as the sunbursts are commonly called. Yet other French researchers determined six periods of time between 1957 and 1958 in which heart attack occurrences rose during peak solar activity and heart failure decreased during low solar activity.[21] This type of research helps prove a theory of geopathic stress; namely, that we are affected by geographic and other energies that interact with the human body.

Intensity Intensity relates to the amount of effort necessary to make something happen. You have to use a lot of effort to create a change on the elemental pathway. The opposite is true on the divine pathway, where you need to accept, not push. On the imagination pathway, you exchange; on the power pathway, you command.

Motion Motion and movement are the same, but there are many factors involved in creating "right motion." Some motions are beneficial, and some are harmful. The four chief ingredients of motion in pathway heart healing are speed, spin, form, and direction. Let's look at each in turn.

- *Speed* is the velocity of energy. Each pathway uses speed a little differently. You usually work with slower speeds on the elemental pathway and faster speeds on the divine pathway. On the imagination pathway, you most often freeze speed and therefore time, and on the power pathway, you control speed through forces.
- *Spin* is the configuration of a moving energy. Spin studies have produced a following among physicists, who are now reading spin to determine the nature of an object and ways to control reality. There are two aspects to spin. In the physical plane, for instance, you might see an object spinning in a circle. When working with some of the other pathways, specifically the imagination pathway, you have to consider the points of the spin that can't be seen when examined normally, within the three dimensions we consciously experience. What might a circular spin look like when seen from the fourth, fifth, or sixth dimension? When observed through a parallel reality or another universe, you might see something entirely different. Through the points that intersect with other worlds, you can gain a perspective helpful for diagnosis or even gather information and energies to enable healing.
- *Form* is the shape energy holds to perform a task. A lot of healers use shapes such as geometric forms, tones, images, and numbers as the basis for healing. Forms are extremely

important on some of the pathways and less vital on the others.

- *Direction* is the goal of moving energy. Determining true direction is vital to pathway healing. You might think you are aiming at health, but what if an internal program is sending energy in the opposite direction?

Charge of Particles Vital to pathway diagnosis and healing on the elemental, the power, and sometimes on the imagination pathway is the determination of particle or wave charge. All particles hold a basic program reflected in the presence or absence of a charge. Protons are positive; electrons are negative; and neutrons are neutral, or absent of positive or negative charges. You will find it beneficial to determine the charge of your primary disease center or presenting malady, as each type of particle carries certain types of misperceptions, feelings, and underlying issues. These components are discussed in chapter 3.

Energy on the Pathways

As stated previously, each pathway is an energetic level of a Greater Reality. I have covered how quantum and other mechanical science ideas, such as using quarks and tachyons, particles and waves, fields and forces, and charged particles can alter energy. You now have the fundamental ideas behind working energetically. In the next chapter, I'll add some important concepts to your healing tool kit, drawing from traditional and alternative health care models and continuing with our discussion of charged particles.

Now let's continue to add to our medical bag with even more knowledge.

chapter three

The Heart of Heart Disease

God creates the cure before He sends the malady.

—Talmud, Zohar i, 196a

If heart disease contains the seed of its own healing, then it would benefit us to understand the disease better. Let's add to our healing tool kit with knowledge about heart disease, from the points of view of traditional and alternative medicine, as well as the Four Pathways approach.

To Know Is to Empower Yourself

If you have heart disease, you owe it to yourself to understand better the nature of your condition. Even if you have already decided to heal yourself in ways more unconventional or esoteric, you would benefit from seeing the "underbelly" of the disease. Knowing how or why you contracted the condition in the first place allows you to better assess the situation for beneficial healing techniques.

In this chapter, we will look at the heart itself and various types of heart problems. I will present the different views of cause, first providing an overview and then outlining several ideas according to traditional, alternative, and pathway models. I will then discuss the most typical solutions, in that same order. Finally, I will offer a brief discussion of the trauma of heart disease, hoping also to energize you for the healing work ahead.

The Heart, as per a Medical Textbook

What's a good physical heart from a medical perspective? Let's examine what the heart does, what it looks like, and how it functions.

Your heart has an awesome task, one that few would accept upon reading the job description. Every day, your heart pumps 2,000 gallons of blood through your body, along 60,000 miles of highways and byways. Whether you are happy or sad, like your life or not, your heart has to keep beating if you are to keep living. It beats about 100,000 times a day; that's about 2.5 billion contractions in an average lifetime.

Physically, your heart isn't all that impressive, but it is busy! About ten ounces in weight, the heart is a muscle divided into four chambers. Blood that has already journeyed through your body is collected in your *veins*. This blood, loaded with waste from the body, is sent into the chambers on the right side of your heart. The upper chambers of the heart are called *atriums* and the lower chambers are called *ventricles*.

The right atrium greets the blood first, then pulses it into the right ventricle. Speedily, the right ventricle passes the blood into your lungs. There, your blood is cleansed of carbon dioxide and enriched with life-giving oxygen. This enhanced blood is delivered to the left side of the heart, first to the left atrium and finally to the left ventricle, from where it is dispersed through *arteries* into your body.

When exiting the left ventricle, your blood enters the body's largest artery, the *aorta*. This artery subdivides like a tree that extends first as branches (*arterioles*), then as twigs (*capillaries*). All of these vessels allow the delivery of nutrients, oxygen, hormones, and other important substances into tissues everywhere. In turn, the blood picks up discarded wastes, toxins, and carbon dioxide and transports them back toward the heart and lungs. Waste products are eliminated through the liver, lymph system, kidneys, bowels, and skin. And technically, your *lymphatic glands* are considered part of your cardiovascular system.

THERE ARE FOUR CHAMBERS IN THE HEART: THE LEFT AND RIGHT ATRIUMS and the left and right ventricles. Blood pumps from the body into the right atrium into the right ventricle, then into the lungs for cleansing and oxygenation. Oxygen-rich blood then exits the lungs into the left atrium, then the left ventricle, where it is dispersed through the aorta into the arteries and into the body. Blood returns to the right atrium via the veins.

Your heart functionality depends on the performance of nearly every other organ and gland in the body. You could consider every cell in the body, in fact, to be a caretaker of your heart. They all receive nutrients and marching orders from the heart and, in turn, offer their own unique gifts to the heart.

Your heart is also a world unto itself. Between each chamber are valves that regulate the pushing of the blood throughout and to and from the heart. These valves must completely close between beats, or blood can pool in a chamber, creating a perilous situation.

The heart muscle itself is called the *myocardium*. It receives its own private supply of oxygen through the *coronary arteries*. These two blood vessels start in the aorta and divide into several smaller arteries.

How does your heart know when and how hard to pump? There are many factors, including a critical one involving electrical energy. Imagine: Every pump of blood must occur in syncopation. The harmony is established by an electrical network of nodes that serve as pacemakers for the heart. These unique cells send electrical impulses to the heart muscle cells and activate contractions. These messages tell the valves when to open and when to shut.

In addition to your electrical system, there is another major player that determines heart health. This is your nervous system. Your sympathetic nervous system can make your heart speed up, while your parasympathetic nervous system can make your heart slow down.

Think of how much exertion it takes to pump the blood hard enough to reach the tips of your fingers and toes. This pumping is measured as your blood pressure. *Blood pressure* keeps the blood circulating in your body. The first factor in blood pressure is the pumping of blood by your left ventricle and the resistance of the arterial channels that disperse the blood. If your heart doesn't thrust intensely enough or if the arterial walls are too wide, your blood pressure will be too low. If your heart pumps too strongly or the arteries are too restricted, your blood pressure will be too high.

The volume of blood moving through your heart also affects blood pressure. Too much blood, and your blood pressure will be too high. Too much pressure and your arteries become damaged. If worked too hard, your left ventricle can become fatigued. Normal or excessive pressure on blocked or weakened arteries can set you up for a stroke or heart attack.

I've barely touched the basics of your heart's work, and already you can see the complications involved in squeezing a single beat from your heart. You can now understand that heart disease is quite complex and can have multiple issues or causes.

When a Good Thing Goes Bad: Cardiovascular Disease

All heart problems fall under the category called *cardiovascular disease*. This is a general term for a collection of diseases and conditions; it is actually not a disease itself. If your doctor says that you have cardiovascular disease, you will want to find out which particular disease or disorder is negatively affecting your cardiovascular system, which consists of your heart and all your blood vessels. Your particular condition will be of two main types:

- Diseases of the heart (cardio)
- Diseases of the blood vessels (vascular)

Some cardiovascular diseases are genetic; you are born with them. These are called *congenital heart diseases*. Others develop later in life from a poor diet, exposure to toxins, or other lifestyle issues. Still other cardiovascular diseases can be caused by other chronic or terminal conditions.

Diseases of the Heart

Here is a brief list of the most common types of cardiovascular diseases (more information is available on MedlinePlus.com, the source of some of this information):

Coronary artery disease (CAD): This is a disease of the arteries that supply the heart muscle with blood. This is one of the more common forms of heart problems and the leading cause of heart attacks. CAD occurs when the coronary arteries have become obstructed and blood flow is therefore restricted. The most typical cause of this blockage is *atherosclerosis*, a form of vascular disease that is usually preventable with proper diet. The word actually means "porridge hardening," or hardening of the arteries. CAD can lead to other heart problems, such as chest pain (*angina*) and heart attack (*myocardial infarction*). A heart attack is actually a problem with the heart muscle, and therefore is considered a coronary heart disease rather than a coronary artery disease.

Coronary heart disease: Coronary heart disease encompasses diseases of the coronary arteries and any resulting complications, including heart attacks, chest pain, and problems with scar tissue.

Cardiomyopathy: This category includes all diseases of the heart muscle. Sometimes cardiomyopathy is genetic, sometimes not. Types include *ischemic*, caused by loss of heart muscle due to a heart attack; *dilated*, or an enlarged heart; *hypertrophic*, in which the heart muscle is thickened; and *idiopathic*, which means the cause is unknown.

Valvular heart disease: This category includes diseases of the heart valves. Damage to the heart valves can lead to narrowing (*stenosis*), leaking (*regurgitation* or *insufficiency*), or improper closing (*prolapse*). Some individuals are born with the disease. Valves can also be injured by conditions including rheumatic fever, infections (*infectious endocarditis*), connective tissue disorders, and certain medications or radiation treatments for cancer.

Pericardial disease: This category includes diseases of the sac, or *pericardium*, that encases the heart. Pericardial disorders include inflammation (*pericarditis*), fluid accumulation (*pericardial effusion*), and stiffness (*constrictive pericarditis*). Some people might have one or all of these conditions. Frequently, these conditions occur after a heart attack.

Congenital heart disease: This category includes heart disorders that develop before birth (they are *congenital*). The most frequent conditions include narrowing of a section of the aorta (*coarctation*) or holes in the heart (*atrial* or *ventricular septal defect*).

Myocarditis: This is typically a viral infection of the myocardial muscle.

Angina: Angina is often one of the first indicators of cardiovascular disease. An angina attack involves a temporary discomfort in your chest, often accompanied by weakness of breath, palpitations, faintness, dull aches in the chest, or sudden pains. It is usually triggered by physical exertion, strong feelings, or sudden stress. Angina most frequently occurs when plaque narrows the coronary arteries, so the blood flowing to the heart cannot supply the heart muscle with the necessary oxygen.

Heart attack: This is a condition in which the heart cannot pump enough blood to meet the need of the body's tissues. It is often called a *myocardial infarction*. The most serious attack is called a *massive heart attack*, caused by a blockage in the coronary arteries.

Sudden cardiac arrest: This is caused by *ventricular fibrillation*, a problem with the heart's electrical system that makes the heart quiver rapidly or erratically. Cardiac arrest occurs without warning and results in a quick loss of consciousness. On the other hand, heart attacks are usually preceded by symptoms.

Heart failure: This condition follows a heart attack. There are three main and often long-term situations that lead to heart failure. These are:

1. The heart beats too fast to compensate for decreased volume or strength.
2. The heart gets bigger to allow more blood to flow through the chambers.
3. The heart muscles thicken to create a more powerful pumping action and move more blood with each beat.

There are two basic types of heart failure. *Acute*, or *sudden, heart failure* results in an immediate failure of the heart to pump the correct amount of blood through the heart chambers. Normally, the heart moves 75 to 80 percent of the blood out of each chamber with each beat. After suffering a critical heart attack, the heart might only move 15 to 20 percent of the blood out of each chamber. The second type includes *chronic heart failure* and *congestive heart failure*. These are ongoing conditions, in which a crippling inability to move blood through the chambers continuously affects the heart. Chronic heart failure often develops over time and is usually linked with salt and water imbalances and kidney malfunctions. *Congestive heart failure* might occur after a heart attack or result from coronary artery disease (CAD). In this case, the myocardial cells are deprived of oxygen, die, and are replaced by scar tissue. The body's tissues don't get needed oxygen and nutrients, which creates difficulty in daily functioning. Blood backs up and veins become overfilled. This excess blood bleeds into the tissues, resulting in lung problems and *edema*, or swelling.

Diseases of the Blood Vessels

Arteriosclerosis and atherosclerosis: Sometimes the walls of the arteries become thick and stiffen, restricting blood flow to the organs and tissues. *Arteriosclerosis* describes this process, and *atherosclerosis* is the most common form of arteriosclerosis. Atherosclerosis refers to hardening of the arteries caused by the accumulation of fatty deposits (*plaques*) and other substances, and it can lead to chest pain (angina) or a heart attack.

High blood pressure: High blood pressure (*hypertension*) is the excessive force of blood pumping through the blood vessels.

Low blood pressure: Low blood pressure (*hypotension*) happens when the heart doesn't pump enough blood intensely enough to assist bodily tissues. This condition can cause atrophy of certain cells and body regions, fainting, and weakness.

Stroke: Known officially as *cerebrovascular accidents* (CVAs), strokes typically involve an *embolism*, or blood clot, and bleeding in the brain. This causes a lack of oxygen to the brain tissue, which kills brain cells. Following a stroke, victims might be paralyzed, weak, unable to speak, or otherwise disabled. Strokes are often linked to high blood pressure. There are many types of strokes. *Ischemic strokes* are silent strokes, and there are two kinds of these. *Cerebral thrombosis* results from a narrowing of the carotid arteries in the neck or the arteries in the brain. A *cerebral embolism* occurs when a blood clot travels from somewhere in the body to the brain, lodges in a brain blood vessel, and cuts off the blood supply to that part of the brain. The major difference between a thrombosis and an embolism is that in a thrombosis, plaque causes the narrowing of the artery. This plaque is localized, and it doesn't move from elsewhere in the body, so the causes are usually atherosclerosis or high blood pressure. There are also *hemorrhagic strokes*, which occur when a blood vessel in or on the brain bursts. This blood then bleeds into the space between the brain and the cranium.

Pulmonary embolism: This occurs when a blood clot travels to the lungs from elsewhere in the body.

Aneurysm: An *aneurysm* is a bulge or weakness in the wall of an artery or a vein in any location in the body. Because aneurysms usually enlarge over time, they can potentially rupture and cause life-threatening bleeding.

Peripheral arterial disease: This is a disorder in which the arteries supplying blood to the limbs—usually the legs—become clogged or partially blocked. When this happens, the arms and legs are left with less blood than they require.

Claudication is pain occurring in your arms or legs during exercise. It's actually a symptom of peripheral arterial disease.

Vasculitis: This is an inflammation of the blood vessels. It usually involves the arteries but may also affect veins and capillaries.

Venous incompetence: With this condition, the blood flows the wrong way in the veins. It most frequently occurs with the stress of infection, inflammation, abnormal blood clotting, or even high-back pressure in pregnancy and can result in varicose veins, skin changes, ulcers, and swelling in the legs.

Venous thrombosis: This is the formation of a blood clot (*thrombus*) in a vein. This clot can damage the vein or break off and travel in the bloodstream. If the clot lodges in the lungs, it creates a condition known as *pulmonary embolism*.

Deep vein thrombosis involves a clot deep within a muscle, such as the calf. Some clots can also cause a stroke.

Varicose veins: With this condition, valves in the veins don't function properly, making blood accumulate in the legs and causing the veins to bulge and twist. The veins appear blue because they contain less oxygen.

Lymphedema: This condition involves an obstruction of the lymphatic vessels, creating a backup of fluid, which can cause swelling and pain. Infections, trauma, tumors, surgery, and radiation treatment may cause it.

Arrhythmia

Another category of cardiovascular disease is *arrhythmia*, an abnormal heart rhythm. This is experienced as a too-fast heartbeat, a too-slow heartbeat, or a missed heartbeat. There are *atrial* and *ventricular* heart arrhythmias, which can be caused by many factors including genetics, allergies, mechanical problems, stress, and scarred heart tissue. They also are sometimes side effects of medications and drugs.

Many arrhythmias are harmless, but there are a few that are especially dangerous. Arrhythmias following an acute heart attack can cause damage to the heart's electrical system, and they must be monitored and treated. Independent of a heart attack, *ventricular tachycardia* occurs when an abnormal electrical impulse coming from abnormal cells in a ventricle makes the heart beat too fast, resulting in an inability of the heart to pump sufficient blood. Ventricular tachycardia can lead to *ventricular fibrillation*, a severe quivering that can cause the heart to suddenly stop. It's one of the most common predecessors of unforeseen fatal heart attacks. Several factors cause arrhythmias: valve disorders, adrenaline rushes, panic attacks, food sensitivities and imbalances, hormonal imbalances, emotional stress, thyroid issues, abnormal mineral levels, the use of caffeine, alcohol, tobacco, and stimulants.

Most people who have experienced heart trouble are frightened of these potentially life-threatening fibrillations. Such fear can create its own emotional stress, which is linked to ventricular problems! In his book *Reversing Heart Disease*, Dr. Dean Ornish notes several studies that show a correlation between emotions and ventricular fibrillation. He also discusses a study by Harvard Medical School doctor Bernard Lown, who recorded that the mere sight of lab personnel can cause ventricular fibrillation in dogs. Dr. Michael Brodsky led another study, as reported in the *Journal of the American Medical Association*, which correlated severe psychological stress with five of six patients who had life-threatening irregular heartbeats.[1]

The Good versus Bad Heart: Caretakers of Your Heart

There are several factors determining the health of your heart. Many of these variables involve structures in the body in addition to parts of your heart.

To really understand the variety of heart conditions in general, and your own in particular, it's helpful to consider the relationship between your heart and other organs in your body, as well as your electromagnetic system.

Your Heart and Other Organs

Your heart relies on a number of organs to carry out its key functions. Your lungs supplement your blood with healthy air and cleanse it of dangerous properties. Your kidneys support the liver and bodily excretion. When the kidneys can't eliminate waste products, toxins back up into the bloodstream and impair all physical processes, including heart function. Kidney imbalance is one of the chief variables leading to congestive heart failure. People with kidney disease are also at higher risk of developing hypertension.

Your pancreas regulates insulin levels, which affect the glucose levels present in your blood, hence the phrase *blood sugar levels*. Hypoglycemia, for instance, is caused by a sudden dip in blood sugar levels; it can cause fainting, weakness, and heart palpitations. Diabetes occurs when your pancreas can't produce enough insulin, and it often creates severe heart problems as the disease progresses.

Your adrenals are also an important part of heart performance. Emitting hormones like cortisol and adrenaline in response to stress, the adrenals can send your heart rate soaring. These surges of hormones are supposed to help you react when in danger, but they can also cause arrhythmia and other heart problems if sustained over too long a period of time.

Even the skin scores a winning point. It is the largest organ in the body; through sweating, the skin releases untold amounts of toxins that, if left in the blood, would dangerously threaten your heart's ability to do its job. The fact is, nearly every bodily organ and gland affects your heart and, in turn, is effected by your heart's processes. If you should study just one organ alone to best understand the heart, however, it would be your liver.

Your Liver and Your Heart: An Old Married Couple?

Your liver and your heart are like an old married couple. If they are engaged in a happy marriage, you'll be happy and peppy. If the marriage is bad, you'll be miserable.

The liver cleanses the body of toxins and wastes. It also manufactures several important compounds that determine the health of your heart. One such substance is cholesterol, which is not a fat, as is sometimes believed. *Cholesterol* is a sterol, a waxy substance essential for good health. It is integral in cell membranes and serves as a building block for cortisone and sex hormones. As necessary as cholesterol is, too much of a good thing causes problems.

There are "good" and "bad" cholesterols. The "good" cholesterol is high-density lipoprotein (HDL), and low-density lipoprotein (LDL) is the "bad" cholesterol. These lipoproteins are spherical particles that carry cholesterol and fat. *Triglycerides* are very low-density lipoproteins (VLDLs). They are fatty acids carried to the liver after eating, and they come from your intestine. HDL is usually able to transport LDL from your arteries to your liver, where it is turned into bile salts and swept out your intestines.

If your body is unable to cleanse itself of excessive cholesterol, your body stores the excess in your bloodstream, usually in the walls of your arteries. The cholesterol buildup is part of a substance called *plaque*. Plaque buildup begins with the passing of LDL through the vessel walls from the blood. Various factors like smoking, high blood pressure, and stress can speed up the oxidation of the LDL in the inner layer of the blood vessel, which causes inflammation and damage to the arterial wall. White blood cells rush to the rescue. Perceiving themselves to be helpful, they gorge on the LDL cells and end up as fatty and foamy cells. Like people who overeat, these overweight white blood cells are unable to move or rid themselves of the LDL. As they die, they give off a fatty porridge that promotes more inflammation.

The smooth muscle cells in the middle layer of the blood vessel attempt to help. Increasing in size and number, they enlarge the arterial walls. *Platelets*, the clotting agents in the blood, also encourage the production of more smooth muscle cells, which then give off collagen and proteins that form plaque. This plaque is called *atheroma*. The situation exacerbates, as atheroma, foamy cells, inflamed cells, collagen, proteins, smooth muscle cells, and cholesterol mix together.

At a more complicated stage, atheromas eventually form into fissures. These interrupt the flow of blood and trigger your body's clotting system. Or the plaque itself ruptures, calling to the site of injury the various ingredients of the clotting process. A collection of platelets, proteins, trapped blood cells, and plaque form a blockage in the artery. This blockage can lead to high blood pressure, in which the heart has to work harder to move the blood around your body. Over time, blood vessels can weaken in reaction, leading to a stroke or heart attack.

It's important to address cholesterol issues on the Four Pathways process, if only because of the physical benefit from having a low LDL and triglyceride count. Sobering research, however, shows that current medical treatments and medicines are not addressing the widespread problem of cholesterol accumulation. Two studies discussed in the same issue of the *New England Journal of Medicine* support this statement. First is a study by the Lipid Research Clinics. Men given cholesterol-lowering drugs had nearly the same number of heart attacks as men given placebos. The other research project, based in Helsinki, revealed nearly the same outcome.[2] On a positive note, in societies in which mean cholesterol counts are 150 or lower without the use of drugs, coronary heart disease is a relatively unknown problem.[3]

Beyond Cholesterol: The Heart Afire

Cholesterol isn't the only measure of a good heart, or a good relationship between the heart and the rest of the body. Anything that causes inflammation in the body will eventually create heart problems. A test called *high-sensitivity C-reactive protein (hs CRP)* is one indicator of systemic inflammation. High CRP levels are associated with a 4.5 greater risk of having a heart attack.[4] Many people now consider the CRP a better indicator of heart problems than cholesterol testing.

Why is inflammation such a critical factor in heart disease? If any part of the body is inflamed, the body's immune system rushes to assist. Sustained and chronic inflammation, often prolonged by long-term infections, emotional or mental stress, or physical toxicity, eventually erodes the immune system, leading to conditions in which the body actually attacks itself. In the case of heart disease, a by-product of a corrosive protein called *homocysteine* is often the culprit, as is a low-grade infection, such as from strep throat, gum disease, or oxidized cholesterol.

Diet and Heart Disease

Your liver will make cholesterol no matter what. Certain people carry genes, however, that tell the liver to produce too much bad cholesterol. Sometimes these genes inflict their message no matter what. Western drugs can be beneficial to these people. Some genes, however, are triggered by environmental, emotional, mental, spiritual, or other energetic factors, from stress to poor eating to the interjection of others' energies. In these cases, it is often helpful to work with Western medicine but also go beyond the norm through the Four Pathways approach. Ultimately, anyone with heart-risk factors must carefully manage his or her diet, as good nutrition will help keep bad genetics under control.

Just as there are "good" and "bad" cholesterol, there are "good" and "bad" fats found in our diet. Good fats, such as vegetable and nut-based oils and the oils found in fish and other oily seafood, can increase your HDL. Saturated fats, which increase your LDL, are found in fatty animal meats and products and high-starch foods containing hydrogenated oils. Over the last few decades, Americans have greatly increased their consumption of bad fats. Cattle, for instance, are now fed grains, which lack the "good" omega-3 fats, instead of grasses. They are also pumped with antibiotics and other chemicals, all of which present a challenge for our body to process.

Studies show that a single high-fat meal will activate the body's clotting mechanism about twelve hours later. As summarized by Dr. Harvey Simon in his book *Conquering Heart Disease*, "It may be that coronary arteries are clogged by clots in the morning because stomachs are clogged by fat the night before."[5]

Another major problem with our diets is lack of nutritional content. In comparison with prehistoric times, which are still the basis of our genetic programming and true nutritional needs, humans once consumed considerably more vitamins, minerals, omega-3 fats, and healthy proteins. On average, for instance, men and women currently consume about 2,500 milligrams of potassium a day, according to the U.S. Food and Nutrition Board. According to Jack Challem in *The Inflammation Syndrome*, our Paleolithic ancestors consumed 10,500 milligrams of potassium a day. Similarly, we now take in 93 milligrams of vitamin C, in comparison with earlier amounts of 604 milligrams a day. Potassium, vitamin C, vitamin E, and all the B vitamins are vital for clearing the body of toxins and preventing inflammation. We have these deficits despite eating more. Recent studies show that 65 percent of all Americans are overweight, of which 31 percent are clinically obese.[6]

We may be eating more, but we're starving for nutrition.

We are also loading our bodies with metabolic disturbances that are poisoning us. Part of the reason that doctors tell heart patients to quit smoking is the amazing amount of toxins found in cigarette smoke, all of which create inflammation in the lungs and the body. There are almost five thousand chemicals in cigarette smoke, many of which release free radicals and other problematic products that damage proteins and accumulate along blood vessel walls.

Another culprit is NSAIDs, a code word for ibuprofen, naproxen, and other over-the-counter anti-inflammatories. Who knew that taking medicine to control a headache might cause a heartache? NSAIDs lower one type of *cyclooxygenase*, an enzyme that converts fatty acids to pro-and anti-inflammatory compounds. But there is a second form of this enzyme, which causes inflammation in the body—and NSAIDS cause your body to produce this second type.

NSAIDs eventually erode the stomach wall. This can lead to something called *leaky gut syndrome*, where the stomach wall thins and allows incompletely digested proteins to enter the bloodstream. These proteins attach to the plaque already formed in blood vessels, increasing clogs and harmful plaque buildup. A recent study found that NSAID use among the elderly with a history of heart disease increases the chances of hospitalization for heart failure by ten times. The two main researchers, physicians John Page and David Henry, concur that use of NSAIDs could account for nearly one-fifth of all hospital admissions for heart failure.[7]

Clearly, heart disease is a complicated set of problems, each of which involves several interdependent aspects of the body. As you proceed through this book, you'll find that the body and physical elements are just the starting point. Your heart is the center of the universe of mind, body, soul, and spirit. The briefest feeling can change your heartbeat. The slightest change in belief can help or harm. This knowledge can greatly impact the way you choose to treat potential or current heart problems.

Diagnosing and Treating Heart Disease: Traditional, Holistic, and Four Pathways Approaches

There are three main categories of approaches for defining the causes and treatments of cardiovascular disease. In general, there is traditional or conventional care, holistic or alternative care, and the Four Pathways system. You will find a lot of overlap between conventional and holistic practices, and probably be astonished to find that the Four Pathways system incorporates both viewpoints and processes. Let's look at the potential causes and treatments from these three points of view.

Potential Causes of Heart Disease: Western Medical Theories

Traditional Western doctors and researchers point the finger at these factors as contributing to heart disease:

- Genetics: Heart disease runs in families. Genes predispose individuals to many factors that can result in cardiovascular problems, including the overproduction of cholesterol, alcoholism, diabetes, adrenal sensitivity, allergies, and hormone irregularities.

- Obesity
- Sedentary lifestyle
- Bad fats
- Cholesterol
- Stress
- Mental factors: Beliefs underlie behavior. Hundreds of studies show that negative thoughts, attitudes, and perceptions can lead to actions that cause heart problems, such as smoking, drinking, and overeating. *You become what you think you are.*
- Hormonal shifts and problems: Women's incidence of heart problems increase with hormonal fluctuations and after menopause. Heart challenges like arrhythmia increase during the period before menopause and during menopause. Stress hormones, including cortisal and adrenaline, also boost the chances of cardiovascular disease by thinning blood vessels, increasing plaque buildup, causing inflammation, and stimulating unhealthy behaviors that are addictive and harmful. Additionally, the hormones and chemicals present in many meat, poultry, and dairy products simulate estrogen, progesterone, and testosterone, creating hormone imbalances that have harmful effects.
- Diabetes
- Smoking
- Alcohol consumption
- Drugs and stimulants including amphetamines, cocaine and other hard drugs, and certain weight loss additives like ephedra change the body's metabolism and can negatively impact many organs, including the heart.
- Gender
- Race
- Age
- Chronic inflammation: Inflammation is part of our body's natural healing process. When we are injured, the immune

system increases blood flow to the impacted area, delivering disease-fighting cells to heal the injury. Continuous inflammation, however, greatly increases the risk of heart disease. Inflamed blood vessel walls attract plaque, inflamed intestines lead to leaky gut, and irritated organs do not function properly. The body even interprets excess weight as inflammation, because body fat, as active tissue, produces hormones that can cause inflammation.

- Allergies: Allergic reactions occur when the immune system attempts to eliminate substances perceived as dangerous to the body. Frequent allergy attacks will lead to chronic inflammation.

Traditional Treatments for Heart Disease

Standard traditional treatment usually involves the following: surgery such as balloon angioplasty, bypasses, cardiomyoplasty, ventricular reduction surgery, radiofrequency ablation, relocation of veins, suturing of valves, valve repair, valve replacement, laser surgery, electrical-node surgery, heart transplant, closing of defects, insertion of shunts or shunt reversals, or electrical cardioversion; certain specialized therapies like thrombolytic therapy, antimicrobial therapy, diuretic therapy, immunosuppressive therapy, or ACE inhibitors; technological aids such as stents, pacemakers and other mechanical pulsing devices, or occlusion devices; a variety of medications and drug treatments, including heart medications, blood thinners, dietary supplements, antioxidant therapy, aspirin, or antibiotics; diet and exercise programs; cessation of smoking, alcohol, stimulants, and recreational drugs; rest; use of supplemental oxygen; treatment of emotional distress; use of techniques for arrhythmias such as Valsalva's maneuver and carotid sinus massage; and other treatments as indicated.

Potential Causes of Heart Disease: Holistic Theories

According to most holistic models, serious diseases like heart disease are caused by mental, emotional, or spiritual factors in addition to physical ones. The holistic construct adds these other factors to those provided under the conventional lists.

- Inaccurate beliefs: We become what we think we are. Countless studies show that beliefs affect behavior. A simple thought like "donuts are good for me" can result in overeating this fatty food, causing a dangerous increase in cholesterol. The belief "I am unworthy" can make us sabotage success.
- Inaccurate ideas about love
- The issues underlying obesity, poor eating habits, use of stimulants, and lack of exercise, which can range from inaccurate beliefs to fear of intimacy and poor self-image
- Unhealthy relationships or relationship patterns
- Repressed feelings
- Hopelessness
- Lack of faith in a Higher Being
- Karma, or problems from the past
- Original sin: God's punishment for others' sins
- Others' energies
- Psychic invasion
- Spiritual choices
- Metabolic disorders caused by inadequate nutrition
- Environmental toxins
- Body imbalances caused by neurological problems or spiritual forces locked into the body
- Vibrational disorders resulting from the long-term effects of geophysical stress, relationship imbalances, negative attitudes, past life issues, among other causes

Holistic Treatments for Heart Disease

Alternative treatments are vast and prolific. They include many conventional treatments as well as adjunctive psychological approaches, including psychotherapy, imagery, group therapy, and support groups; macrobiotics; nutritional-metabolic programs, including various diets, supplements, and herbal treatments; traditional Chinese medicine; religious, energetic, and spiritual healing; technological treatments, including use of computers, radionics, light frequency, and vibrational technologies; electromagnetic therapies; psychic treatment; homeopathy and other vibrational medicines; manipulative treatments such as chiropractic and massage; folk and shamanic treatments; exercise and breathing techniques; and other treatments as recommended by a holistic practitioner.

Potential Causes of Heart Disease: Four Pathways Approach

There are so many potential factors in the Four Pathways approach that I can't list them all. The reason the Four Pathways system is called an approach, however, is that you can easily approach diagnosis and therefore healing in a few simple ways. Most healing on the Four Pathways involves diagnosing through the chakras and invoking specific properties of each Pathway. All heart disease can be sourced to a chakra because chakras carry all the information concerning bodily conditions. Each operates like a computer networked into a mainframe computer. Just as a virus on a single computer can compromise an entire computer network, our body can be only as healthy as each of the chakras. Because the data controlling each chakric area is shared throughout the overall system, a harmful belief, feeling, spiritual idea, or physical condition in one area can affect all other areas—thus, it is possible to trace a heart problem to a chakric area far from the heart. Furthermore, a problem with the heart chakra can create a malady elsewhere.

Throughout this book, you will continue to learn how the chakras serve as doorways to the Four Pathways. You will learn more about the roles of the chakras in causing and healing heart disease in chapter 4. For an explanation of how chakras can create heart trauma, see "Chakras and Vibrational Information" in chapter 4.

The following are fundamental factors that cause heart disease for each pathway:

Elemental Pathway: Unbalanced positive and negative energies and the misperception and vibrational energies that keep these in a stuck and reinforced pattern.

Power Pathway: Misapplied powers and forces or lack of knowledge of how to command healing forces to make changes.

Imagination Pathway: Misperceptions that make us think we don't have choices. Healing is stuck on the "other side" of reality, and we continue to hold on to heart disease in "this reality."

Divine Pathway: Perceptions that keep us cloudy and unable to recognize or fully embrace the power of divine love.

Healing Actions through the Four Pathways Approach

As described in this book and *Advanced Chakra Healing*, healing processes include:

Elemental Pathway: Shifting of particles and waves; release of interference; searching for causes in multiple spacetimes; use of symbols, colors, shapes, and tones; dealing with feelings, beliefs, or other fixations; working with kundalini, elements, pH balance, nutrition, diet, exercise, and other body needs from an energetic perspective; working with aspects of self; ultimately, attaining a neutral state through the chakras and other energy bodies.

Power Pathway: Shifting and enhancing spiritual energetic forces through the chakras.

Imagination Pathway: Shifting energies from the antiworld to this world and vice versa, through the center of a chakra; use of symbols to hold new changes; ultimately, achieving a neutral space within a chakra center so you can make healing decisions.

Divine pathway: Activating a spiritual wave or quality of Truth that combats one of the seven major "lies." Ultimately, accepting divine love and grace.

Benefits and Potential Problems: Traditional, Holistic, and Four Pathways Approaches

In order to safely choose among processes, it is best to look at the benefits and potential problems of conventional, holistic, and Four Pathways care.

Benefits and Potential Problems of Traditional Care

Today's cardiologists are hopeful. They believe recent advancements in coronary health care can lead to the reversal of heart disease. Their newest regimen includes high-powered lifestyle changes, use of new surgical techniques and technology, high doses of cholesterol-lowering drugs, a new form of dialysis to cleanse the blood, and bypass surgeries that include the intestines. While we await these fresh and exciting treatments and findings, we must continue to work with conventional treatments. The current methods would not be available if they were not effective some of the time. A responsible patient conducts his or her own research on new, alternative, and emerging treatments while simultaneously making the best use of treatments that are well-established.

One of the major current treatments is the regimen of cholesterol-lowering drugs. A very real problem with this course of treatment is the cost of these drugs, as well as their side effects. Common secondary effects include nausea, bloating, pain, weakness, and intestinal and libido problems. As stated by Dr. Dean Ornish in his book *Reversing Heart Disease*, only two studies to date have shown that cholesterol-lowering drugs may reverse heart disease, and even then only in a minority of patients. Yet another study done by the National Heart, Lung, and

Blood Institute determined that these drugs did not reverse coronary heart disease at all![8]

Other studies suggest that cholesterol-lowering drugs, most of which are "statin drugs," can actually harm the body and be a factor in heart disease. To reduce the production of cholesterol, they inhibit an enzyme called HMG-CoA-reductase. Turning off this enzyme erases its availability for the needed production of estrogen, testosterone, and corticosteroids.

As pointed out by Jack Challem in his book, *The Inflammation Syndrome*, another disadvantage of statin drugs is that they inhibit the body's use of coenzyme Q10, or CoQ10. One significant side effect of lack of CQ10 is muscle weakness. The heart muscle contains the largest amount of CQ10.[9]

Even short-term use of statin drugs or corticosteroids, another set of commonly prescribed anti-inflammatory drugs, can create ongoing heart problems. Although these drugs are used to reduce inflammation, they can also cause inflammation by wiping out healthy bodily functions and interfering with the absorption of key metabolic substances, including folic acid, potassium, zinc, vitamin D, calcium, and the B vitamins.

Many people believe that taking a pill does the job, but the only true reversal of heart disease universally seen has been accomplished through major lifestyle alterations, including change of diet, supplementation of healthy for unhealthy fats, and exercise. This statement does not preclude surgery and the use of life-supporting technology and medications at least for the short term, which are necessary to deal with crisis and stabilize the body.

Medications for high blood pressure are as equally suspect. Again, they are costly and their results are questionable at best. In one study conducted by the National Heart, Lung, and Blood Institute, 43,000 patients with hypertension were followed for about five and one-half years, and blood pressure drugs did not significantly reduce coronary mortalities.[10]

There are other issues regarding the use of medications to regulate heart disease. First, if the heart is interdependent with other organs, we must consider the damage medications cause these secondary organs. The liver incurs problems with the heavy use of medications, especially those directed toward it. If the liver can't clean the blood or properly regulate HDL cholesterol, aren't we creating two monsters where there was once a single one? Second, medication can often mask other symptoms and problems. Side effects cause very real physical reactions. We need to ask which ones indicate a medication issue and which ones should be linked to the heart ailment or some other disorder.

Obviously, using surgery, implantations, and even medication can be life supporting. The key problem with relying only on traditional care is that you may never get to the bottom of the real heart problem, which could lie in a different organ or in an emotional, mental, relational, psychic, or spiritual issue. Many physicians now believe that heart disease might mainly stem from stress, but what can they offer the patient? As shared by Dr. Bruno Cortis in his book *Heart & Soul*, approximately 75 percent of all health problems come from stress, and the most devastating types of stress are psychological and emotional.[11] Cortis actually believes heart disease to be a disease of loneliness and difficulty in sharing oneself with others.[12]

Surgery can save a life, but can it address deeper issues of isolation? Medication can control your heart rate, but can it prompt intimacy?

Diet and exercise can eliminate unhealthy fats and strengthen your cardiovascular system, but can they alone unleash subversive, life-threatening feelings? Traditional health care is necessary, but it is incomplete.

Benefits and Potential Problems of Holistic Care

Alternative medicine accounts for some of the greatest gains in heart treatment over the years. Now, even traditional medical doctors recommend supplementation of diets with folic acid, omega-3 fats, CoQ10, antioxidants, grape juice, and certain herbs, all thanks to the persistence of the holistic community.

Cardiologists may or may not eagerly embrace some of the less standard protocols of alternative methodologies, though studies show their effectiveness. Making lifestyle changes has become an obvious task for healing, and several studies emphasize this observation. One of the reasons I recommend the protocol by Dr. Dean Ornish is that his lifestyle recommendations are backed by scientific research. For instance, in a clinical study, 82 percent of patients who made his recommended lifestyle changes, including increased exercise; prayer or meditation; reduced consumption of trans fats, red meat, sugars, and caffeine; and increased mineral-rich foods that contain good fats, demonstrated measurable reversal of coronary artery blockage within one year. In contrast, the majority of the heart patients who followed their doctors' advice became measurably worse during that same amount of time.[13]

Dr. Ornish also speaks to the importance of dealing with emotions, mental stress, and spirituality, an area more typically accentuated by holistic rather than conventional practitioners. A proponent of decreased isolation, Ornish defines isolation as separation from our feelings, from our inner self, from others, and from a higher source.[14] Studies support Ornish's prescription for healing heart disease. Consider a study conducted at the University of Michigan for over a decade. During those ten years, two-and-a-half times more men who didn't participate in altruistic volunteerism died than men who performed volunteer work.[15] Social connections and spiritual purpose affect how we live—and if we live!

Mental stress can also play a big part in heart problems. Two researchers, Dr. Andrew Selwyn of Harvard Medical School and Dr. John Deanfield at the Hammersmith Hospital in London, scanned subjects' hearts while they were doing easy mathematical problems. The stress of this simple undertaking measurably reduced blood flow to the heart.[16]

Prayer has consistently been a source of healing and inspiration for religious people. Studies are showing that prayer can benefit heart patients. Consider, for instance, a study reported in

2001 undertaken at Duke University Medical Center, in which cardiac patients who received intercessory prayer as well as coronary stenting had better clinical outcomes than those receiving standard stenting treatment alone.[17]

The main problem with holistic care is that it is scientifically difficult to support. There are few studies showing the effectiveness of holistic medicine. Holistic medicine is not a regulated field, and few people are aware that there are actual dangers in alternative treatments. It's fine to take low doses of vitamin E for your heart, but did you know that it is an anticoagulant? The uncontrolled nature of the holistic field could create a disaster for uninformed patients.

It can also be challenging to pinpoint the exact cause of a disorder. Do you know whether a particular feeling, belief, spiritual issue, or physical disorder, or all of the above, causes your heart issue? Even if you can pinpoint the general nature of the cause, how do you go about narrowing your search further? Consider a feeling-based heart disease. Which of the dozens of feelings you experience every day are causing you grief? Of these feelings, at what age did they become troublesome? Are these feelings even yours? You can absorb feelings that aren't your own, and these can be at the root of all your problems, not just a heart crisis! Alternative medicine can be a rich source of help, but it can also be overwhelmingly complicated and cumbersome. A qualified practitioner is a must, and a treatment plan that doesn't counteract traditional treatments is a requirement.

Benefits and Potential Problems of the Four Pathways Approach

The chief challenge to the Four Pathways system is that it is new. There are no studies showing its effectiveness, merely anecdotal evidence. There aren't pathway doctors, and so you face the same challenges as you would if working conventionally or holistically. You must find and evaluate your own professionals. However, the Four Pathways system does incorporate both conventional and holistic wisdom, so you can choose the best of all worlds. It also places you in charge of your own process.

The most useful aspect of the Four Pathways system is that it is chakra-based. Chakras provide an access method that is physical and spiritual, present-oriented and futuristic. By working with the chakras, you can actually get to the bottom of a disorder, then shift precise energies for healing. In summary, the Four Pathways approach:

The Four Pathways system allows you to attain the ultimate healing space—the Greater Reality, the place in which you are already whole and healed.

- Embraces the best of traditional care
- Upholds the ideals of holistic medicine
- Can be worked simultaneously with traditional and holistic methods
- Boosts the gain of traditional and holistic treatments
- Becomes increasingly less complicated as you rise through the pathways
- Offers choices in care and supports personal responsibility
- Costs little to no money
- Causes maximum impact through the Four Pathways connections
- Works on the energy of the situation, the pivot in making a difference
- Creates change where it matters
- Assumes wholeness, therefore potentially allows healing to occur miraculously
- Has no negative physical side effects, and alleviates the negative side effects of other treatments

Pathway healing supports conventional medical care, yet proposes the use of other methods to counterbalance negative side effects.

There is much to be gained by the healing ahead, which begins—and ends—with the chakras.

chapter four

Shifting through the Chakras

The universe is change; our life is what our thoughts make it.
—Marcus Aurelius Antonious, *Meditations*, iv.3

Your chakras are your portals to the Greater Reality, and the Four Pathways get you there. Your chakras are similar to elevators in a large downtown department store in that they operate between the various levels of reality composing the greater whole. If you want to journey to the land of the "nines," you enter the ninth chakra of any of the four pathways and slip easily from floor to floor, or in this case, from pathway to pathway. To address issues governed by the "ones," you voyage through the first chakra on any of the pathways.

While elevators traditionally operate only vertically, in the human body you can also travel horizontally from one chakra to another. The second chakra links the first and the third, and so on. You can also connect through the myriad of other energy bodies found on the different pathways. Let's examine these energetic elevators more completely, taking the ancient knowledge of chakras to a whole new level of healing.

Endless Wheels of Light

The word *chakra* comes from a Sanskrit phrase meaning "spinning wheel of light." There are twelve basic human chakras, seven of which are in the physical body and emanate from your spine, where they spin in a vortex fashion front and back.

From the elemental pathway to the divine pathway, each pathway "adds" a component to a chakra, making them extremely powerful forces. On the elemental pathway, a chakra is a medley of fundamental units, such as carbon and oxygen, sodium and potassium, ions and electrons, tachyons and quarks. On this level, chakras look like alchemical soups of spirit and matter. On the power pathway, a chakra appears as a circular band of moving forces. On the imagination pathway, a single chakra condenses to a mirror, a place of choice. With a thought, you can flip the patterns and problems of this reality for the possibilities and programs of another reality. On the divine pathway, a chakra transforms into a burning channel of pure light. Here, healing is simple. Love "unbends" the "crooked" light that creates disease in the physical body. Love "straightens you out," so your light flows evenly again. Immediately, the chakra blessed on the divine pathway transfers its healed state throughout all four pathways, and the body is healed. The main vehicle for this process is the chakra system.

No matter which pathway you work with, the inherent wholeness and health of your Greater Self emerges and invites healing.

Chakras are often called subtle energy bodies, because they vibrate at speeds and in spins that are difficult to perceive with the physical eye. Dr. Richard Gerber, author of *Vibrational Medicine*, asserts that "subtle energies at the etheric level are merely at a higher octave than the physical."[1] As previously explored, your chakras work differently on each pathway but only in terms of vibration, substance, or degree of frequency. On every pathway, they work energetically and manage the same basic life concerns.

Most healers, wise people, and sages perceive the chakras psychically. Modern science is beginning to substantiate the existence of chakras and auric bands. Consider the work of Dr. Valerie Hunt of Stanford University and author of *The Science of Human Vibrations*. Together with healer Rosalyn Bruyere, this scientist pioneered audiotapes and other evidence of the seven major chakras, showing the different tones, and measures of frequency, among the chakras.[2]

Tones are only one way of distinguishing the frequency differences of the chakras. Many psychics discern differences in the chakras by color; others, by sense or feel. In general, the lower the chakra, the lower the vibration; the higher the chakra, the higher the vibration. The heart lies in the center of the twelve-chakra system, merging the infrared energies of the lower scale with the ultraviolet frequencies of the upper scale.

Chakra Basics

Here is a table of the primary location of each chakra, its vibratory color, and its overall purpose. My book, *New Chakra Healing*, provides additional information.

Chakra	Location	Color	Overall Mission
First	Genital area	Red	Security and survival
Second	Abdomen	Orange	Feelings and creativity
Third	Solar plexus	Yellow	Mentality and structure
Fourth	Heart	Green	Relationships and healing
Fifth	Throat	Blue	Communication and guidance
Sixth	Forehead	Purple	Vision and strategy
Seventh	Top of head	White	Purpose and spirituality
Eighth	Just above head	Black	Karma and universal linkages

Ninth	A foot above head	Gold	Soul programs and plans
Tenth	A foot below feet	Brown	Legacies and nature
Eleventh	A film around hands, feet, and body	Pink	Forces and energy conversion
Twelfth	Around the body and thirty-two points in the body	Clear	Ending of human self, access to the energy egg

Chakras and Vibrational Information

Fundamentally, chakras are communication organs of light. Each regulates a different set of physical, emotional, mental, and spiritual concerns, as well as relational and psychic data. Chakras operate on information and vibration, or informed vibration. A specific chakra will attract, decode, interpret, encode, and disseminate information that matches its information base or particular vibration.

A chakra isn't much different than a physical organ, except in one major area. Your physical organs work only with sensory information—quarks, which travel slower than the speed of light. A chakra does the same, but it can also process psychic information—tachyons, which jet about faster than the speed of light.

A chakra actually has two parts, a front and a back. The front regulates conscious and daily concerns, while the back works with unconscious and historical issues. Chakras look like two black holes meeting at the small end, and in fact, the comparison of a chakra to a black hole does not stop here.[3] The chakra holds a conical shape and processes light, absorbing some light into itself and emanating some light outside of itself. Based on its programming, the chakra is able to attract certain types of informed vibration, as does a gravitational black hole. The chakra can work with photons or energies that are virtual—unreal, psychic, invisible, and inaudible—and make them real, and vice versa. And the chakra does this within a spacetime that is fluid; that is, it changes on an as-needed basis.

However, a chakra has an advantage over a black hole in that it has two sides. Hence, you achieve a constant *exchange* of informed vibration from the unconscious and historical to the conscious and everyday. You can insert a "desired future" through the front side, and create the future in front of you through one of your paired virtual photons. You can unearth a bit of knowledge from the past in the back of a chakra and pass this knowledge into your current life through the front of the chakra.

Think in terms of your heart, the meeting center of all energies. There is a horizontal exchange, but also a vertical one. Through the heart center, you can transmit spiritual truths from above and affect the physical condition of your body through your lower chakras; you can also make behavioral changes through your lower chakras and emanate new spiritual truths through your upper chakras. Through the heart, you can do all things.

This cross-dimensional nature of the chakras is also responsible for the multiple causes of heart disease. A disturbance in any chakra can create a heart condition. Following is a chart outlining the various body parts managed by the twelve major chakras. I'll be drawing upon this information to explore the ways that energy from many areas can create—and heal—heart disease.

Chakras in the Physical World

This chart lists the physical body parts and functions governed by each chakra.

Chakra	Physiological Locations
One	Genital organs and endocrine system; coccygeal vertebrae; affects some adrenal, kidney, bladder, and excrement functions
Two	Intestines; part of the adrenal endocrine system; parts of kidney function; some aspects of reproductive

	system; sacral vertebrae and the neurotransmitters determining emotional responses to stimuli
Three	Pancreas endocrine system; all digestive organs in stomach area, including the liver, spleen, gall-bladder, stomach, and parts of the kidney system; lumbar vertebrae
Four	Heart and lungs; circulatory and oxygenation systems; breasts; lumbar and thoracic vertebrae
Five	Thyroid endocrine gland; larynx, mouth, and auditory systems;lymph system; thoracic vertebrae
Six	Pituitary endocrine gland; parts of the hypothalamus; parts of the visual and olfactory systems (including the left eye); memory storage
Seven	Pineal endocrine gland; parts of hypothalamus; higher learning and cognitive brain systems; parts of the immune system and brain glands affecting moods, emotions, and hormones
Eight	Thymus (immune system); memory retrieval functions; aspects of the central nervous system; the right eye
Nine	Diaphragm; pineal gland; corpus callosum and other higher learning centers, including the cortex and neocortex
Ten	Feet, legs, and bones
Eleven	Skin and muscles
Twelve	Secondary chakric sites—there are more than thirty-two located throughout the body, including the knees, elbows, palms, and internal organs

A Multiple-Choice Test:
Primary Disease Sites of Heart Disease

Chakras store all the data you've ever generated in relation to that chakra's area of expertise. This means you can access your chakras to discover the core cause of a heart disorder.

Not all heart diseases are caused by an imbalance in the heart chakra. Consider the adrenals, a first-chakra organ. Adrenal stimulation can force cortisol into your body. One long-term effect of this first-chakra activity is increased inflammation and the buildup of plaque. As shown in a study by Dr. Ilan Wittstein of Johns Hopkins, any sudden stress or trauma, such as the death of a loved one or a car accident, results in symptoms identical to a heart attack, including similar EKG readings. For the people in this study, adrenaline levels shot up thirty times higher than normal.[4]

Even the higher, spiritual chakras can come into play. Many forms of depression, for instance, are regulated by the seventh chakra, which houses the pineal gland. Studies, including one at the University of Birmingham in England, show that depression doubles an otherwise healthy person's risk of a heart attack.[5]

In pathway healing, you benefit by working directly with the chakra that hosts the cause of the heart problem. Therefore, all pathway healing begins by locating the *primary disease chakra*, the chakra holding the cause of the problem. There may also be a *secondary disease chakra*, which might hold secondary causes or serve as the chakra that acts out the problem. If adrenaline is the primary cause of the presenting heart condition, we would say the first chakra is the primary disease chakra and the heart chakra is the secondary disease chakra.

Often, the primary and secondary sites will be the same on all pathways. If the first chakra is causing the problem, you would focus healing energy on the first chakra and then, after that, on the heart chakra. If you can't determine whether a non-heart chakra is involved and you have a heart condition, you can simply focus your work on your heart chakra.

As your own pathway healer, you can work with vibration instead of, or in addition to, information in order to conduct diagnosis and healing. Chakras can vibrate "out of tune" or "in tune." The presence of a disease process creates great disturbance in a chakra's vibration. You can therefore use methods such as psychic hearing, toning, pendulum, and other techniques suggested throughout this book to work with your primary and secondary disease chakras. A healthy tone matches the frequencies of your own harmonic, which you are guided to discover in chapter 7. The most discordant chakra will probably be your primary disease chakra. When performing healing work, you might also want to determine your most attuned chakras; you can shift healing energies from them into their handicapped chakra cousins.

Searching for Harmful Vibrational Information

The most effective strategy for healing heart disease is to think in terms of patterns. All heart ailments stem from a *pattern*, or a repetitive behavior or model. If your heart skips once in a while, you're okay. If your liver emits high cholesterol in response to a rare indulgence, you're not in any grave physical danger. If your adrenals get a little overwrought once in a while, you'll be fine. If you repress anger so that you don't get fired, you're being smart. If these or other underlying causes of heart disease occur on a regular or overly frequent basis, though, you will develop a pattern, and patterns lead to problems.

Internal and external negative behaviors can culminate in heart problems because they disrupt your natural, personal harmonic. Any time you create a chronic vibrational disturbance in the body, physical ailments will occur. A certain set of vibrational disruptions will lead to heart disease rather than other maladies; this depends upon frequency of behavior and your personal susceptibility. If you disturb your heart's vibration too much, you will gradually alter the information that keeps your heart healthy.

When a vibration is disturbed, the information is altered. Consider substance abuse. If you drink too much alcohol, over time you disturb the harmonic of your liver, which becomes unable to access the genetic codes or chemical messages that regulate cholesterol. Your liver is now misinformed and because it is operating with a lack of necessary data, it cannot properly cleanse your blood and perform other tasks critical to maintaining a healthy heart.

You might ask, How am I ever going to discover what is causing the "disturbance in informed vibration" responsible for my heart disease? Remember, the clue lies in your primary disease chakra. The beauty of working with chakras is that by locating the chakra that's causing the greatest disturbance, you can unlock the physical, mental, emotional, spiritual, psychic, or other factors creating illness.

Finding the cause isn't as complicated as it sounds. Only three types of information are communicated through the chakras. There is *useful information*, which assists and sustains you in meeting your life purpose. This data supports health. There is *neutral information*, which doesn't do much of anything. Neutral information doesn't hurt you; neither does it serve you. Then there's *harmful information*, which is detrimental to achieving your spiritual mission and can actually create disease and poor health. When looking for the cause of heart disease, you must separate harmful from useful or neutral information. Harmful information is what underlies patterns, in the form of faulty programming.

There are two basic types of programs. A *program* is a code that establishes choices and decisions. There are good programs and bad programs. Good programs create good habits, which are healthy responses to life; bad programs form patterns, which are automatic reactions. Although there are some positive patterns, most automatic responses are detrimental. A reaction that works in one situation doesn't necessarily assist in a different one. Your healthiest programs involve the *original programming* of your inner spirit. This programming is your spirit's master code, which directs the chakras to select information telling you what to do, how to feel, and what to think. You are a spiritual being, and your spiritual perfection is programmed into every chakra, every cell, and every aspect of your being. You are already whole, and buried within your chakras is the programming for wholeness in health and well-being.

If chakras were allowed to develop and operate without intervention, you'd be healthy most of the time. You would intuitively process only useful information and discard what is meaningless or harmful. Your physical system would constantly attune to your spiritual dynamic and would easily achieve homeostasis, internal and external balance or coherence. Unfortunately, this isn't an ideal world. Chakras are altered by life experience. Just as they can store and operate on information that is life sustaining and joyful, so can they hold and serve data that supports dysfunctional beliefs, unhealthy behaviors, and illness.

A chakra can store a lot of negative data, created as a result of bad programs. Bad programs can affect any or all aspects of your being, including physical, emotional, mental, spiritual, relational, and psychic. Not all bad programs result in heart disease, but there are certain types that do, especially those that have issues of love at their core.

It's important to understand bad programs, for repairing or rewriting them is the basis of Four Pathways healing. In everyday life, your psyche continually merges beliefs and feelings to form *emotions*, or "e-nergy" in "motion." Emotions motivate or move you to action. Spy a man in a leather jacket with a gun in a back alley, and you're out of there! You run because the feeling of fear partners with the belief that "guns are dangerous," and your nervous system says, "Take flight!" When that feeling and belief are permanently paired in a way that causes harm, your fearful reaction doesn't get turned off. Then, if your six-year-old holds a squirt gun in the air, you might jump ten feet! Or perhaps you forged the belief that someone in a leather jacket should be feared, and you won't ever talk to men in leather jackets. Emotions should disband after they are used, or they become bad programs instead of helpmates.

Another word for a bad program is a *stronghold*. There are two basic types of strongholds. An *emotional stronghold* joins a belief and a feeling, whereas a *mental stronghold* cements two or more beliefs. The leather-jacketed thief is an example of an emotional stronghold. An example of a mental stronghold is the marrying of a belief like "milk is good for you" with the idea that "you should always eat what's good for you." And what if you're allergic to milk? You'll be sick!

Strongholds underlie patterns, and no one wants to get stuck in a ritual that holds them hostage. Perhaps your blood pressure rises because of a mental stronghold that creates a physical pattern: you believe that "good people should suffer" and that "you will get lazy if you don't put 'pressure' on yourself." The result? To be a "good person" you take jobs that you hate and force yourself to work hard. The resulting stress raises your blood pressure. An emotional stronghold can just as easily result in an adverse pattern. Perhaps you were raised to believe that "anger is bad" and that you'd be punished by God if you expressed your anger. The resulting fear, coupled with the belief that anger is bad, is enough to send anyone's adrenals, therefore heart rate, skyrocketing whenever anger is present—your own anger or someone else's.

Strongholds often lurk under the bad behaviors that precede heart disease. Obesity, lack of exercise, smoking, use of alcohol or drugs, and overeating of sugars and trans fats are leading factors in heart disease. You can overeat to repress your feelings, stay fat because of fear, smoke to hide from intimacy, abuse drugs because you think you're bad, and watch television all day because you believe you have nothing to offer the world. There is no limit to the strongholds that can develop into nasty, disease-producing patterns.

Patterns appear differently according to each pathway. Elemental patterns are endless in number, and can include just about any physical, mental, emotional, or spiritual factor. Power patterns are force-based; here you will search for causes that are supernatural. On the imagination pathway, a pattern reduces to a choice—what made you choose the reality of heart disease versus a potentially different reality? Through the divine pathway, heart disease is an invitation, not a pattern; it is a call to love.

Diagnosis and Healing: The Basics of Informed Vibration

Every heart problem reduces to negative, positive, or neutral energies, or a mixture. Positive-based heart conditions express anxiety and mental strongholds. Negative-based heart issues involve depression and emotional strongholds. Neutral-based heart problems reflect a core misperception, usually regarding love. The easiest way to conduct pathway healing is to establish the percentage of negative, positive, or neutral energies causing your heart condition. This knowledge will influence elemental pathway treatment, power pathway forces, imagination pathway choices, and divine pathway perception that can invite recovery. Following is a description of each of these informed vibrations as they appear in my mind's eye. You might want to read these lists quickly now, then refer back to them after reading the Special Insert: Pathway Ideas and Techniques, which explains concepts such as working with colors, tones, symbols, inference, and energetic contacts.

Positive-Based Cardiovascular Conditions

- The coloration will be yellow, discolored yellow, or off-white.
- Coloration when healing or healthy will be gold or white.
- The primary disease chakra or the physical disease site will psychically look like swirling or spinning areas of yellow or yellow-white energy; if you analyze the information in these areas, you can determine the nature of the spiritual misperception creating the discord.

- The patient will tend toward anxiety and express fears about the future.
- Affected chakras will spin too fast and move clockwise.
- In general, positive-based illnesses will originate in the second, fourth, sixth, eighth, tenth, and twelfth chakras.
- Positive-based heart conditions will create or be caused by an alkaline imbalance.
- Elementally, there is usually too much water and other yeast-, fungal-, or bacterial-producing elements in the body.
- Managing energy bodies, the energy organs of the elemental pathway, are disconnected from each other.
- The auric field is too thin.
- Coloration of affected chakras is too light.
- Tones of affected chakras are too high.
- Symbols will tend to be circular but will be broken or misshapen, or energetically connect the patient to bad sources.
- Symbols reflecting the heart problem will reveal issues with self-love and will indicate a tendency to use love to avoid personal power.
- The main issue to uncover is spiritual; healing must provide new data to change the vibratory rate into the correct harmonic.

Neutral-Based Cardiovascular Conditions

- Coloration is red or a discoloration of red, such as muddy red or brick red.
- Coloration when healing or healthy will be pink or rose.
- Primary disease chakra or illness site will psychically look like red material standing out on a flat plane. You might find cordage, such as life-energy cords, leading into the stricken area.
- Patient is apathetic, non-nurturing, and confused.

- Affected chakras don't spin, or they move very little.
- Any chakra can be affected.
- Neutral-based heart conditions create both acidic and alkaline imbalances in various parts of the body.
- Elementally, there is almost always too much metal present (to serve as protection), which can also create heavy-metal toxicity in the body.
- Feelings are nonexistent or hard to discern.
- The heart chakra will reflect few or no connections to anything, anyone, or any time period. This situation reflects the patient's tendency to be unable to move forward or backward in life or to grasp love.
- Auric bands lack intensity and fluidity; they are stuck in one position.
- Tone of affected chakras will be flat and lack pitch and depth.
- Symbols will be of one variety and extremely fixated. They will not move or flow.
- The system will not have a variety of numbers; everything will be the same.
- The main issue to uncover is love; power issues are secondary. Somewhere along the line, the patient fell out of love with him- or herself—and life. The other major issue is a fear of personal power, which is the right to claim your place in world. Essentially, the patient needs to learn how to vibrate with life energy so as to give and receive love.

Negative-Based Cardiovascular Conditions

- The coloration will be dark blue or murky black.
- Coloration when healing or healthy will be a strong black or silver.
- The primary disease chakra or illness site will psychically appear as blobs of ugly blue or black material; if you assess the information within, you will uncover psychic or physical

toxins; repressed feelings or parts of the self; cords and other energetic contracts and various forms of interference.

- The patient is depressed, despairing, and stuck in the past.
- Affected chakras spin too slowly or move counterclockwise.
- The majority of chakras bearing negative-based illnesses are usually the first, third, fifth, seventh, ninth, and eleventh chakras.
- Negative-based heart conditions will create or be caused by an acidic imbalance.
- Elementally, there is usually too much fire and other viral-inciting elements in the body.
- Managing energy bodies on the elemental pathway are too connected with each other; there is a lack of independent functioning.
- Feelings are depressing, causing sadness and rage; feelings may not be one's own but could be interjected from others.
- The patient's issues are rooted in the past; there is a lack of release from prior situations.
- Auric field is too thick or murky.
- Coloration of the affected chakras is dark, heavy, and blobby.
- Tones of the affected chakras are too low.
- Symbols will tend to be boxy but will be too thick, broken, misshapen, or misused. They will indicate cords or other energetic connections to interference.
- Symbols indicating the heart condition will reflect mis-understandings about the use of power and will reveal a tendency to become powerful in order to avoid confronting intimacy issues.
- The main issue to uncover is power; healing must focus on vibrating the energies so as to access information that can be used for personal empowerment.

Working the Chakras at the Source

Working with informed vibration is so beneficial that I always assess a heart patient for the presence of negative, positive, or neutral energies. When you have just one primary disease chakra and it is primarily a single energy, your diagnosis and treatment can be pretty uncomplicated. Consider working on the elemental pathway in this case. With a negative heart chakra, for instance, you might immediately search for repressed feelings, energetic contracts (see the Special Insert for more information), psychic and physical toxicity, and lingering issues from the past. If the heart chakra is primarily positive, concentrate on spiritual misperceptions, fears of the future, and the presence of fungus or bacteria. For a neutral-based heart chakra, focus on the fact that an entire life is based on a giant falsehood or a misperception about love. Find the lie and you can exchange it for truth.

Typically, a heart condition will present a blend of the three types of informed vibrations. You may also be faced with more than one disease site. My advice is always to begin and end your work in the primary disease site. Start at the source of the problem and the secondary problems will be much easier to address.

Connected Heart: The Heart's Many Helpers

Several factors determine the health of your heart. Many of these variables involve structures in the body in addition to your heart.

To understand the variety of heart conditions, and your own in particular, it's helpful to consider the relationship between your heart and other organs in your body, as well as your electromagnetic system. Each organ is linked to a specific chakra, therefore the first step in pathway healing is to determine which chakra might be causing the type of heart problem you intend to treat.

Chakras and Affiliated Heart Conditions

It is implied that all heart conditions can be primary to the heart chakra, therefore I have not listed any cardiovascular diseases under the heart chakra except those involving organs besides the heart, such as the lungs.

You will also notice a considerable list under the first chakra. The first chakra regulates blood and the circulatory system, so it is a primary factor in many cardiovascular conditions.

First Chakra

When working with the first chakra, you will want to concentrate on survival and security issues. The first chakra influences life energy, the basic energy that keeps us alive. All life-threatening cardiovascular conditions require work in this chakra.

Cardiovascular Condition	Additional Chakras Involved and Special Notes
Coronary artery disease	Other chakras can be involved, especially the third
Coronary heart disease	Other chakras can be involved
Cardiomyopathy	(Also eleventh chakra)
Varicose veins	(Also tenth chakra)
Peripheral arterial disease (PAD) and claudication	(Also tenth chakra)
High or low blood pressure	If the "pressure" is security-oriented (also tenth or eleventh chakra)
Chronic heart failure	If involving kidneys or primary fears (also second or third chakra)
Massive heart attack	Involves subconscious decision to end life, or indicates someone or something emanating a strong desire for your life to end
Sudden cardiac arrest	Linked to unconscious issues affecting electrical system. These issues can be internal or external. External can involve sudden shock, death wish from others, or even entity attacks (also tenth chakra).
Angina	Involving sudden threat. Other chakras can be involved.

Electrical and magnetic-based cardiovascular issues	(Also sixth and seventh chakras)
Arteriosclerosis and atherosclerosis	(Also second or third chakra)
Valvular disease	
· *Stenosis*	Fear of passion of life choices; insufficiency indicates lack of life energy.
· *Prolapse*	Equates to fear of personal identity or commitment to life. Other chakras can be involved.
Pericardial effusion, as well as the other pericardial diseases	The pericardial mirrors the womb and holds in utero issues
Coarctation	This congenital narrowing of the aorta indicates lack of belief that life will hold the full self (also tenth chakra)
Arrhythmias	Due to electrical or magnetic safety issues or issues locked into the subconscious or the unconscious. The latter can affect the electrical or magnetic energies of the heart and can be caused by internal issues or external factors, such as a catastrophe or attack from an entity.
Aneurysm	For secondary causes
Vasculitis	For secondary causes
Venous thrombosis	For secondary causes
Cardiovascular problems	From adrenal stress
Cardiovascular disease	Related to overconsumption of red meat
Cardiovascular disorders	From addictions related to hard drugs, alcohol, and other dangerous metabolic disturbances
Cardiovascular conditions	Stemming from abusive or harmful sexual activity, such as being the victim or perpetrator of sexual abuse; also diseases resulting from contracted sexual illnesses, such as AIDS

Second Chakra

Many second-chakra conditions start with repressed, unexpressed, or judged feelings or emotional strongholds (the latter would cause a pairing with the third chakra). The feelings causing a disease might not be your own. I believe that up to 80 percent of the feelings causing physical or life disruptions have been absorbed from someone else. Someone else can also hold one of your feelings, leaving you with an empty space and the inability to access or express a feeling necessary for self-care or survival. You must evaluate whether a feeling is yours, using techniques in the Special Insert in chapter 5.

Cardiovascular Condition	Additional Chakras Involved and Special Notes
Chronic heart failure	If involving kidneys or issues of repressed feelings or creativity (also first or third chakra)
Angina	Involving emotional issues. This is a primary source of angina. Other chakras can be involved.
Coronary artery disease	From emotional repression. Other chakras can be involved.
Arteriosclerosis	From emotional rigidity (also first and third chakras)
Atherosclerosis	From repressed emotions (also first and third chakras)
Valvular disease	Especially mitral valve prolapse in women along with first chakra, representing fear of feminine power and identity
Arrhythmia	From repressed feelings
Cardiovascular diseases	Caused or affected by hormone changes or fluctuations, as in many arrhythmias
Cardiovascular diseases	Due to emotional issues
Cardiovascular issues	Related to the colon, as in poor digestion, leaky gut, and more
Cardiovascular issues	Related to dietary allergies and addictions involving "sticky" carbohydrates, such as gluten and wheat, yeast, and milk products

Third Chakra

In working the third chakra, you want to search for mental strongholds, and perhaps emotional strongholds, in concert with the second chakra.

Cardiovascular Condition	Additional Chakras Involved and Special Notes
Chronic heart failure	If involving kidneys or issues of inaccurate beliefs, such as those causing low self-esteem (also first or second chakra)
Thrombosis	When caused by atherosclerosis, as well as chakra localized to the clot
Angina	Involving negative thoughts. Other chakras can be involved.
Coronary artery disease	Involving issues with third-chakra organs, such as liver problems that result in atherosclerosis or hardening of the arteries. Other chakras can be involved, such as the first.
Arrhythmia	From self-defeating beliefs. Other chakras can be involved.
Atherosclerosis	Due to plaque buildup managed by the liver and beliefs leading to emotional repression (also first and second chakras)
Arteriosclerosis	From beliefs leading to emotional rigidity (also first and second chakras)
Cardiovascular issues	From disturbances with digestive organs, including liver issues, cholesterol buildup, food allergies, diabetes-related disorders, hypoglycemia and other blood sugar problems, and insulin challenges
Cardiovascular issues	Resulting from addictions to alcohol, consumption of sugar, and overuse of caffeine, artifical sweeteners, or colas

Fourth Chakra

All cardiovascular problems will involve the heart chakra. Cardiovascular diseases affecting the heart can also involve the following issues:

- Relationship discord
- Addictions related to alcohol, primarily wine or wine coolers
- Addictions related to the lungs, such as smoking or sniffing any hard drug, such as cocaine
- Food allergies or addictions to sugar or chocolate
- Lower heart issues, such as the core self based in fear or shame instead of love and truth

Fifth Chakra

Fifth-chakra heart issues always concentrate on communication issues or interference that alters one's natural communication processes.

Cardiovascular Condition	Additional Chakras Involved and Special Notes
Arrhythmias	Caused by thyroid imbalances and being critical
Cardiovascular conditions	Caused by the following: • repression of one's truth, views, and needs (front issue) • nervous eating • cords and other bindings forcing negative beliefs (back issue)
Lymphedema	Refusal to release your own or others' energies, feelings, or psychic energies
Myocardial infarctions	Caused by entity attacks on the soul. Other chakras can be involved.
Angina	Caused by criticism from living or nonliving sources. Other chakras can be involved.
Cerebral thrombosis	From a narrowing of the carotid arteries
Ischemic strokes	These are silent—what aren't you hearing or saying?

Sixth Chakra

The core of all sixth-chakra heart disorders lies in self-image distortions, which, in turn, affect hormonal and other regulatory factors.

Cardiovascular Condition	Additional Chakras Involved and Special Notes
Arrhythmia	Involving the hypothalamus and self-image issues (also seventh chakra)
Electrical and magnetic-based cardiovascular issues	(Also first and seventh chakras)
Cardiovascular disorders	Caused by pituitary-controlled hormones, as in menopausal fluctuations in women or decrease in human growth hormone in both genders
Angina	Involving hormonal fluctuations
Strokes	Other chakras can be involved
Cardiovascular issues	Resulting from self-image issues or problems, such as anorexia, bulimia, or other food issues

Seventh Chakra

Almost all cardiovascular diseases would benefit from working with the seventh chakra, the body's home for the spirit, especially if positive-based heart disease is involved.

Cardiovascular Condition	Additional Chakras Involved and Special Notes
Strokes	Most cerebral embolisms and hemorrhagic strokes, as a secondary site. Other chakras may be involved.
Arrhythmia	Involving the hypothalamus (also sixth chakra)
Cardiovascular conditions	Can be caused by symptoms involving anxiety, depression, lack of spirituality, meaninglessness, lack of purpose, or overuse of stimulants or artifical sweeteners

Eighth Chakra

Eighth-chakra heart issues often originate in the past—your own or some-one else's. Grasp the right to break free from the past, and you empower yourself for healing.

Cardiovascular Condition	Additional Chakras Involved and Special Notes
Venous incompetence	Inability to separate past from present; could also be caused by exchanging others' energies for your own
Congenital heart problems	As in those carried over by a past life
Cardiovascular diseases	Caused by past-life issues or sorcery
Myocardial infarctions	Involving entity or black magic attacks. May involve other chakras.
Angina	Involving entity problems. May involve other chakras.
Arrythmia	Involving entity attacks or fears from past lives
Atrial or ventricular septal defect	These "holes in the heart" often stem from past-life situations
Strokes	Involving past-life issues
Cardiovascular illnesses	Caused or supported by lifestyle choices used to increase one's shamanic or mystical powers, such as addictions to sugar, coffee, caffeine, alcohol, and sex

Ninth Chakra

Does idealism interfere with your own health? This is the core misunder-standing underlying ninth-chakra heart problems.

Cardiovascular Condition	Additional Chakras Involved and Special Notes
Angina	Involving worry about the world. May involve other chakras.
Arrhythmia	From inordinate guilt
Sudden strokes	If guilt is involved
Cardiovascular diseases	Taken on to "help the world," such as through guilt or shame in being blessed

Tenth Chakra

Nature can heal—or harm. An imbalanced relationship with the natural world or the people who came before us creates tenth-chakra cardiovascular problems.

Cardiovascular Condition	Additional Chakras Involved and Special Notes
Genetically based (congenital) cardiovascular diseases	Involves issues carried in by own soul or current lineage
Diseases induced from environmental toxicity	Repression of tenth-chakra gifts (environmental and natural psychicism) or emotionally charged reactions to nature (i.e., an emotionally traumatic incident occurred in spring, resulting in allergic reaction to pollen)
Myocardial infarctions	Involving security issues. Can also stem from energetic attacks from family members or ancestral hauntings. May involve other chakras.
Coarctation	This congenital narrowing of the aorta indicates belief your family can't accept the real you (also first chakra)
Varicose veins	Can indicate resistance to living grounded in body (also first chakra)
Peripheral arterial disease (PAD) and claudication	Can indicate resistance to bringing earthly energy into body (also first chakra)
High or low blood pressure	If the "pressure" is family-based (along with fourth and potentially first or eleventh chakra)
Valvular disease	Due to childhood illness, such as rheumatic fever. May indicate inability to filter the issues and needs of others due to soul patters. May involve other chakras.
Sudden cardiac arrest	Due to subconscious soul or family issues affecting the ventricular system. Can involve attack from ancestral

	haunting or family member's energy (also first chakra).
Angina	Involving familial issues or attacks. Can involve other chakras.
Arrhythmia that is genetic (i.e., inherited inability of heart to process potassium)	Caused by ancestral issues
Cardiovascular conditions	Caused by familial or ancestral interference or attachments that run in the family

Eleventh Chakra

Do you know you have the right to command forces for well-being? Do you know how to do it ethically and safely? These are the issues involved in eleventh-chakra heart problems.

Cardiovascular Condition	Additional Chakras Involved and Special Notes
Myocardial infarctions	When involving loss of positional or personal power. May involve other chakras.
Coronary heart disease	When scar tissue or heart muscle issues are involved
Cardiomyopathy	Ask who or what is "putting the squeeze" on you, making you expand beyond what is normal, or making you lose power (also first chakra)
Many valvular diseases	Usually indicates difficulty maintaining personal boundaries
Deep vein thrombosis	Indicates deep self-loathing, rejection of power
Angina	Involving issues of powerlessness
Arrhythmia	Involving misuse or lack of ownership of power
Cardiovascular problems	Caused by issues of powerlessness or inability to command for personal needs, such as high or low blood pressure

Twelfth Chakra

Heart problems originating here involve issues about connection. The twelfth chakra is most frequently a secondary site, and should be addressed when cardiovascular disease caused by organisms that affect twelfth-chakra areas (such as virus or bacteria that injure the heart, blood vessels, and the twelfth chakra-related joints) is present.

Cardiovascular Condition	Additional Chakras Involved and Special Notes
Valvular heart disease	Especially those involving connective tissue disorders. May involve other chakras.

A Special Note

Remember that every cardiovascular disease will have either a primary or a secondary site in the fourth chakra. The heart controls the circulatory system and focuses energetically on relationship and love. You should always work with the heart chakra in some capacity if you have either a cardio or a vascular disease.

Vascular diseases are more likely to involve the fourth chakra and at least one additional chakra. Vascular disease of the veins and arteries, such as PAD, nearly always establish themselves in the legs. The legs are centered between the tenth and the first chakras, and conditions in this area might involve both chakras. A general rule of thumb is the closer the clot or condition to the ground, the more apt it is to involve the tenth chakra rather than the first chakra. Thighs in general store issues from our mother and father, so they are usually first chakra based, as are maladies involving the hips. In the case of a disease like pulmonary embolism, which involves transfer of a blood clot from perhaps the legs to the heart, you are dealing with two primary disease sites. Lungs are essential to the fourth chakra, and they regulate ideas and emotions about grief. A clot that begins in the calves, for instance, will probably equate to a tenth- and fourth-chakra issue; one that originates in the thigh area will merge the first and fourth chakras.

Certain chakras store the energies creating a disease in a site or an organ associated with that chakra. As pointed out, legs can hold issues of the tenth or first chakra; however, the heart uses several receptacles to preserve its basic integrity from harm. Shoulders, elbows, wrists, and knees are typically holding vehicles for heart issues.

Some cardiovascular diseases can involve nearly any chakra. Myocarditis, for instance, is caused by a viral infection of the myocardial, or heart muscle. Here, I would deal with the fourth chakra but seek the origin of the virus. Viruses indicate that something outside your energy system is trying to control you. They can involve an attachment to a group consciousness, such as a family of origin belief system, a genealogical ideal, a cultural or religious group, or a past-life soul group. Strep infections, for instance, can lead to heart damage. Strep occurs through the mouth or fifth chakra; therefore I would seek a viral cause in this area. Certain sexually transmitted diseases can hurt the heart; for example, syphilis weakens the heart muscle and almost all herpes and chlamydia organisms damage the circulatory system over time. For these, I would work with the first chakra. Types of arthritis can injure the heart. What was the entry point of the arthritis? If it's the joint, consider adding the twelfth chakra to the list of disease chakra sites.

Arrhythmia can have many origins. The tenth chakra regulates the subconscious, as does the first chakra, which also operates a major part of the unconscious. The ventricles hold our subconscious issues; the atrium, the unconscious. Hence, a ventricular fibrillation will probably involve the tenth or perhaps first chakra; an atrial condition such as atrial tachycardia, the first chakra. However, the second chakra can initiate an arrhythmia if repressed emotions are involved; the third chakra, if you're working with negative beliefs and poor digestion; the fifth chakra, if you've repressed so many words they have "landed" in your heart, where they cause disturbance; the sixth chakra and seventh chakra, in that these manage brain patterns; the eighth chakra, if you've carried over a past-life issue; the ninth chakra, if you feel guilty about not helping the entire world; the eleventh chakra, if you can't claim your own power and so you disempower your own heart; and the twelfth chakra, if you've made poor connections with other people.

You also can analyze for location in the matter of diseases like strokes, vasculitis, and aneurysms. A thrombosis is a localized clot, and it usually affects the area it is housed in. This localization allows you to assume that the primary chakra site is within this geographic area. Other strokes occur from traveling clots, such as with cerebral embolisms, and you must source the origin of these clots to assess for primary cause. Aneurysms can bulge in almost any artery, although there are favorite spots, and vasculitis also affects mainly the arteries but sometimes the veins. Again, turn to the physical location to determine the primary disease chakra.

You will also notice that the first chakra comes into frequent play. The first chakra regulates the blood and circulatory system, issues of safety and security, and your basic electrical and magnetic systems (the latter is also regulated by the fourth, sixth, and seventh chakras). If you are dealing with life-and-death issues, you should consider working with the first chakra, along with any other presenting diseased chakras, if for no other reason than to establish your right to life before working deeper. A little detective work can go a long way.

chapter five

Intuition: Tools for Energy Mapping

To understand reality is not the same as to know about outward events. It is to perceive the essential nature of things.

—Dietrich Bonhoeffer, *Ethics*†

Many people fear their most important healing tool: intuition. Intuition can be a proverbial double-edged sword. It cuts through to the essential nature of things.

When you use your intuition to open the windows of your heart, you also open your heart's healing powers.

The Key to Shift Healing: Using Your Intuition

Intuition is the conscious use of your inner psychic abilities. Access your intuition and you can diagnose illness, perform healing, energy map, and shift between pathways.

In this chapter, I'm going to briefly describe intuition. You'll then take the "Psychic Style Quiz," which will help you determine your own innate intuitive gifts. As you read through the descriptions of the various intuitive styles, you'll gain insight into how you can best apply your intuition to your heart-healing process.

†Bonhoeffer, Dietrich, *Ethics* (New York: Touchstone, 1995), p. 70.

This chapter also includes a special section describing various energy-healing tools.

The Intuitive Advantage: Gaining the Edge on Healing

Intuition is versatile. Depending upon its application, you can use it to unearth the issues causing a heart problem, select the most effective technique for healing, and shift energies between pathways.

Intuition is applied psychism. You are innately psychic. Everyone is born able to communicate psychically, which simply involves communicating with fast-moving information-energy. When information travels faster than the speed of light, it seemingly breaks natural law. You can predict the future, erase the past, know what your friend had for dinner, and even communicate with someone a thousand miles away. You can know what is seemingly unknowable—like the nature of a heart condition or the process that might provide healing.

Each chakra hosts a distinct psychic ability. Some of your chakras' psychic gifts are stronger than others, as they are vital to your spiritual destiny. The gifts in other chakras might be physical in nature, or esoteric, involving hearing, sensing, or seeing the invisible.

We are psychic because psychic abilities assure our survival. Unfortunately, most adults have lost touch with their abilities, usually because of fear or lack of support. People often fear that which empowers, and your psychic qualities can empower you to make effective, personal, and spirit-based decisions. Claim your psychic strengths and you own the ability to transform your life into a testimony of health and wellness.

Developing Your Intuition

It's important to spend time in developing your psychic talents. The hidden world is full of helpful information, energies, and assistants. It also comes complete with negative or nonapplicable information, energies, and dissuaders.

Psychic abilities are natural but raw. You have to understand, manage, and mix them intelligently to reach a desired goal. You wouldn't grab any old ingredients out of the refrigerator and throw them together when making a cake, would you? No, you'd want to follow a recipe—that is, if you want a cake rather than a stew. Part of the psychic development process involves analyzing the programs that tell your chakras how to use their psychic abilities. Programming from the following sources can affect psychic abilities positively or negatively:

- childhood experiences
- parents and extended family
- ancestral beliefs and traditions
- peers
- schools
- religious institutions
- the media
- your community
- the culture at large
- your soul and spirit
- the Divine
- the world of spirits

Ironically, these innate psychic gifts can actually be a source of cardiovascular disease! The psyche has few, if any, boundaries. Without boundaries, the energetics of someone else's problems, illnesses, issues, beliefs, or feelings can enter you. What is not yours to process cannot be processed in your body, and it turns into psychic, and eventually physical, toxins.

Psychic data can originate in the past, present, or future, and this data can create stresses that can, in turn, cause heart problems. Memories (either yours or someone else's) can lock into your body, creating a primary disease site. Current situations can hit you out of the blue—literally penetrating your skin, stimulating a stress reaction such as heart palpitations, liver malfunction, sugar cravings, or an adrenal flush. These energies might only temporarily damage the body, but if your reaction turns into a pattern, it can create long-term injury. Even knowledge from the future can generate heart trouble.

Research is now supporting the fact that many people are affected negatively by psychic abilities. Consider a startling project conducted by researchers McCraty, Atkinson, and Bradley for the Institute of HeartMath in Boulder Creek, California, and the Institute for Whole Social Science in Carmel, California, as published in the *Journal of Alternative and Complementary Medicine*. The participants in the study were shown thirty calm images and fifteen emotionally provocative pictures. The heart rates of a significant number of the participants responded to the emotionally charged images even before seeing them. The study suggests that the heart receives future information before our senses perceive it, allowing us to prepare for events before they begin. Interestingly, the women in the study were more responsive to this intuitive information than the men. Apparently, both the brain and the heart receive the intuitive stimulation, but the heart actually collects and responds to it first![1]

I have found that the best way to prevent negative psychic input is to first separate positive from negative beliefs; to assess which psychic gifts to use, and how; and to establish intuitive boundaries. The following are a few pointers.

Intuitive Healing Requires Boundaries

Take your innate psychic gifts, add boundaries and parameters, and you've created intuition. Intuition is psychic ability used consciously and safely. *Boundaries* is a psychological term that refers to the need to be safe. Your front door is a *sensory boundary*. It keeps people out, unless they are welcome. *Psychic boundaries* screen physical energy but also emotional, mental, and spiritual energies. They assure security at all levels.

Psychic parameters are less strident than psychic boundaries. If a boundary is like a door or a wall, a parameter is equivalent to a guideline or a standard. A parameter gauges information-energy that attunes to your personal harmonic, or real self. A parameter can perceive which parts of an energy, a thought, an emotion, a person, or an idea fits for you, and which parts don't, and invite only that which fits into your energy field.

In pathway healing, a honed psychic ability or intuitive faculty allows you to transfer energy from place to place and release energies causing problems. Intuitive faculties enable you to tap into sources from the following eight major *levels of psychic sources*:

1. The physical world, including animals, plants, elements, and spirits of nature
2. The emotional plane, including feelings and emotions from other people and entities
3. The mental plane, including thoughts, beliefs, ideas, and fears from other people and entities
4. The relational plane, including anything or anyone, alive or dead, to which you have a bond or connection
5. The energetic plane, the world in which all energy interacts, also containing the beings that attend these processes
6. The soul plane, which involves all communication between your soul and those of others
7. The world of spirits, which includes all spirits, alive or dead, positive or negative
8. The world of the spirit, the base of which is the Divine

These sources vary in availability and helpfulness from one pathway to another. Your intuition is vital for accessing sources and establishing boundaries and parameters. Several types of invisible sources are described in the Special Insert in this chapter, and I have highlighted certain sources for each pathway in the individual chapters for each of the pathways. As you apply your intuition in pathway healing, you will find it becomes available for everyday life, as does your link to the spiritual dimensions.

Sympathy versus Empathy

What's the main difference between being psychic and being intuitive? It's the use of *sympathy* versus *empathy*.

Sympathizers often take on external energies. You can actually absorb energies through your skin and into your organs. You cannot process energy that is unlike your own. Unlike information disrupts the information and vibration of your own system and can cause organic damage, as well as electrical disturbances.

Some gurus, religious figures, and healers use sympathy as a healing tool, such as that involving the process of transmission. *Transmission* is the full transference of energy from being to being. You can allow transmission if it follows the rigors of the divine pathway and involves the selfless giving of unconditional love.

Empathy involves registering rather than assuming energy. Empathizing is much safer than sympathizing. When you register energy, you keep its charge outside of your body. This way, you can perceive or "read" the information, but your personal harmonic isn't barraged by frequencies that can throw you off balance.

Psychic Style Quiz

What are your most appropriate and keenest intuitive gifts to use for energy mapping? This quick quiz will give you a start on the answer; a more complete test is available in *Advanced Chakra Healing*.

Directions: Please respond to the following questions by selecting the most applicable number. A "0" indicates you've never experienced this phenomenon; a "5" indicates that you experience the phenomenon constantly.

1. I sense others' physical conditions in my own body.
   0 1 2 3 4 5

2. When I'm at the movies or reading a book, I feel the characters' experiences in my own body.
   0 1 2 3 4 5

3. I always know what others are feeling emotionally.
   0 1 2 3 4 5

4. I am like a human sponge for others' emotions.
   0 1 2 3 4 5

5. I often know information I've never been taught.
   0 1 2 3 4 5

6. I sense, in my stomach, whether or not someone is being honest.
   0 1 2 3 4 5

7. I easily predict the outcome of peoples' relationships.
   0 1 2 3 4 5

8. I often find myself helping people with their relationship concerns.
   0 1 2 3 4 5

9. Words will come to me as soon as I open my mouth.
   0 1 2 3 4 5

10. I can hear words, tones, or guidance from beings that aren't present.
    0 1 2 3 4 5

11. I often get information via pictures in my mind.
    0 1 2 3 4 5

12. I get visions that tell me what to do.
    0 1 2 3 4 5

13. It's easy for me to sense right from wrong.
    0 1 2 3 4 5

14. I sense what the Divine plans are for myself or other people.
    0 1 2 3 4 5

15. I have always been able to enter a trance state and connect with different worlds.
    0 1 2 3 4 5

16. I remember having been alive before, and I can sometimes see others' past lives.
    0 1 2 3 4 5

17. I am naturally concerned about the global impact that actions might have.
    0 1 2 3 4 5

18. I seem to know what's going on in others' souls.
    0 1 2 3 4 5

19. I know myself as one with nature.
    0 1 2 3 4 5

20. I get my guidance and energy from the natural world.
    0 1 2 3 4 5

21. I can command energies and forces to do my will.
    0 1 2 3 4 5

22. Through my hands and feet, I can move energy at my own bidding.
    0 1 2 3 4 5

Scoring, Part I: Add your total scores in each of these areas:

Questions 1 and 2
Questions 3 and 4
Questions 5 and 6
Questions 7 and 8
Questions 9 and 10
Questions 11 and 12
Questions 13 and 14
Questions 15 and 16
Questions 17 and 18
Questions 19 and 20
Questions 21 and 22

These numbers could indicate strong or weak tendencies in each of the eleven major psychic styles, according to these divisions:

Questions 1 and 2	Chakra One, Physical
Questions 3 and 4	Chakra Two, Feeling
Questions 5 and 6	Chakra Three, Mental
Questions 7 and 8	Chakra Four, Relational
Questions 9 and 10	Chakra Five, Verbal
Questions 11 and 12	Chakra Six, Visual
Questions 13 and 14	Chakra Seven, Spiritual
Questions 15 and 16	Chakra Eight, Shadow

Chakra Psychic Gifts

Here is an overview of the types of gifts innate to each chakra. I explain each psychic gift, then add advice on how to use this ability in an intuitive fashion. Additionally, I offer counsel on using this gift to energy map and shift heart disease.

Chakra one: Physical sympathy. You are a very physical person and in touch with what is going on in your own body, as well as in the material world. Unfortunately, you can absorb others' illnesses and make them your own. If you have heart disease, ascertain whether you have taken on someone else's heart problems, either the physical condition or the emotional, mental, or spiritual issues that increase the propensity for heart problems. One of your psychic gifts is the ability to perform *psychometry*, or reading information stored within physical objects. To use this gift for diagnosis or healing with heart disease, hold a pendulum (such as a stone on a necklace) over your fourth chakra. Next, determine whether a clockwise swing indicates a "yes" or a "no" by asking your name. Then ask questions such as these: Did this heart problem originate with me? If not, did it come from (fill in the blank)? If the root cause of the heart disease lies outside of you, query how best to free yourself. You can also test the validity of an herb, a supplement, or a treatment modality using this technique. If you don't have a pendulum or it would be awkward to use one at a given moment, you can distinguish answers and choices by your body's reactions to statements. A true statement or supportive choice will "feel good," and a false statement or unsupportive choice will "feel bad."

Chakra two: Feeling sympathy. Feeling-oriented, you easily take on others' feelings. Check to see whether any aspect of a heart problem is caused by others' feelings or your vibrational sensitivity to them. When internalized from other people, feelings can't be processed physically and often end up stored in the heart, where they cause energetic obstruction and eventually physical blockage. Feelings can also be held within or attached to all sorts of other elements, including food, air, and power pathway forces. Certain heart conditions can result from reactions to these feelings. To compensate, use your sensitivity to feelings to help you diagnose and heal from feeling-based problems. How do you feel when you eat certain foods? Associate with specific people? Positive energies will leave you happier and lighter, those to reject will cause depression or anxiety. Use the exercise "The Transpersonal Process" in the Special Insert to release others' feelings from your body.

Chakra three: Mental sympathy. You are *clairsentient*, which means "clear sensing." This means you constantly gather and organize psychic input in the forms of thoughts, ideas, and facts. What a useful tool for the heart patient or healer who wants to uncover the root cause of a heart condition or assess the pathways for supportive measures! Sometimes your sympathetic gift is your undoing, however. Gathering information that fails to align with your natural self can create confusion, mental disorder, and bad behavior—like eating too much sugar, using too much caffeine, or overworking, the types of activities that lead to heart problems. Begin assessing information through your solar plexus. What data "feels" accurate? What causes your "stomach to turn"? A useful exercise is to picture a yellow fishnet around your entire third chakra area. Ask the Divine to program your third chakra so that you input information that betters your health and reject information that is unhealthy. Every morning, reaffirm the presence of this filter so you remain strong and clear all day long.

Chakra four: Relational sympathy. You are the relationship maestro of the chakra system! Heart-based people are also the healers of the chakra zodiac, constantly wanting to help fix other people. You can't help someone else by assuming his or problems or by over-worrying. In fact, these are two of the major energetic causes of heart disease. Apply your sensitivity wisely by determining whether your heart problems are, in part, due to these factors: overbonding, caretaking, a closed heart, self-protection, assumption of another's issues or healing needs, lack of self-love, or the inability to give or receive love. A key healing technique is to allow the Divine to open, cleanse, and heal your heart. Open the back of your heart chakra to bring through divine love and heal you from the inside out.

Chakra five: Verbal sympathy. You are gifted in *clairaudience*, which means "clear hearing." This ability involves receiving psychic data as tones, verbal messages, or written messages. The key to good health is to make sure you are sourcing helpful energies or entities. Do this by setting clear parameters and boundaries or by calling on a gatekeeper—an angelic or spiritual being who acts as your "stop sign." Avoid the worst of the *transmediumship* gift, which involves allowing external energies into your body, by *channeling* or listening only to the wisdom, diagnostics, or healing energies acceptable to your gatekeeper or your own spirit. Increase your healing powers by using verbal commands on the power pathway to heal concerns. Words and tones can also summon healing energies on any of the pathways.

Chakra six: Visual sympathy. You perceive psychic information in pictures, symbols, colors, or shapes. Called *clairvoyance*, or "clear seeing," this gift is perhaps the most reliable for energy mapping and diagnostics. You can view images within your head or draw them to illustrate the origins of disease; vibrational qualities of the causes of a heart problem; and energies, colors, tones, or elements that will heal. Ask to see through your higher self or spirit for best results.

Chakra seven: Spiritual sympathy. The most spiritual of the chakras, your seventh center invokes the power of *prophecy*, the gift of knowing what is destined or fated. Learn how to mediate, pray, or visualize through your pineal gland, the contact point of the seventh chakra, to determine the reasons you have a heart condition. As you concentrate on this part of your brain, ask yourself questions like these: Is your heart problem helping you learn a spiritual lesson? If so, what? Is there another way to garner this learning? Does your heart problem involve a mis-understanding, a mistake, or an illness assumed from someone else? The pineal gland is one of the main links to the world of spirits and the Divine. Connecting first to the Divine, ask to know consciously how to heal your heart. Allow the grace of the Divine to show you the way.

Chakra eight: Shadow sympathy. Do you know what a shaman is? Those gifted in the eighth chakra stand midpoint between the worlds, dimensions, and planes of existence, mediating infor-mation from one place to another. This job can put a great strain on the physical body, and more so the heart, the center of the energy system. Learn to use your shamanic gifts for your own benefit. Read the *Akashic Records*, recordings of all that has ever occurred, and look for curses, bindings, and other control tech-niques. You can work with any of the pathways to search for truth and healing, but perhaps you will excel on the imagination path-way. Enter an altered state before working.

Chakra nine: Soul sympathy. As someone devoted to ideals, you excel at working with higher principles and can invite physical reality to conform to these ideals. Some soul sympathizers, how-ever, take on others' soul issues because of a misguided sense of love, and others assume the ills of the world, making their own heart sick out of concern for others. Work on the power pathway to command energies to adapt to the highest plan. In addition, use your gift to read the language of souls. Within the ninth chakra lies all the knowledge needed to learn about your own or another's soul identity, plan, symbols, desires, and relationships. Check whether cords, curses, and other energetic contracts compromise any of your gifts.

Chakra ten: Natural sympathy. Nature is alive with energies, spirits, and truths for healing. You are innately capable of hearing, sensing, feeling, or seeing into the heart of anything natural. Watch your tendency to assume the pain of the planet. Instead, learn to read the signs of nature as shamans do, looking to animals, planets, and plants for diagnosis. Then, on the elemental pathway, use the properties of nature for healing, whether through diet or divining. Call upon energies such as elemental beings or faery helpers to assist you, and reach into the power pathway to infuse your work with supernatural forces. You can learn how to accept the properties or nutrients of anything in nature directly into your body for healing and information.

Chakra eleven: Force sympathy. The eleventh chakra connects with the eleventh auric band. Through this chakra you receive knowledge of the forces that might be keeping you ill or those that can provide healing. Through this auric band, you command movement of these and other forces to meet your goals. Practice using the elements, spirits of the elements, and spiritual energetic forces of the power pathway for your own healing.

Continuing to Develop Intuition

Here are some methods to further transform your psychic abilities into intuitive faculties.

Cultivation: Take classes, read books, and practice in daily life. If you feel blocked, work with a spiritual director or a psychotherapist, as trauma can sometimes block our gifts.

Prayer: Prayer is talking to the Divine. The act of reaching for the Divine opens our own divinity. Once we are receptive to the messages and love of the Divine, we paradoxically strengthen our healthy psychic boundaries, assuring safety.

Meditation: Meditation invites divine response. A calm mind is more receptive to the awesome messages of the Divine, which are often packaged in commonplace, everyday events. If you ask a specific question, you may not obtain a reply during your meditative practice, but you will at some point receive an answer.

Contemplation: Contemplation involves enjoying the presence of the Spirit. Love heals all, and love is everywhere. This healing presence automatically smoothes your chakras and auric field.

Intensity: Pay attention to your strong inspirations or gut senses. The more powerful the message, the greater likelihood it is important. If you receive advice three or more times, either psychically or in daily life, heed the wisdom. Psychic information sent or received in a highly emotional or spiritual state is more likely to attract attention. Use this knowledge in reverse, and intensely communicate your needs to others and the Divine when you are ill, or if you want to receive attention. You will be heard.

Religious or spiritual study: Study after study shows that people are more likely to receive spiritual revelation if they believe in the Divine, by any name. The type of psychic phenomenon noted fits with cultural and religious icons.

Desire: Do you really want something? Notch up your desire to 110 percent, and your desire can be fulfilled. The second and sixth chakras are involved in manifesting, as the feelings from your second chakra instruct your sixth chakra to open to an infrared energy that can transform spiritual reality into physical matter. Simultaneously, your seventh chakra can pull physical energy upward from your first chakra and spin your sixth-chakra desires into the universe. Mean what you say, say what you mean, and act accordingly.

Illness: Don't be dismayed if you are learning about your intuition for the first time while you are ill. Use your illness. Strong sensations, including pain, fear, and suffering, force us to reach beyond the bounds of the five senses. It's actually easier to tap higher brainwaves or achieve an altered state of consciousness when ill. Go into your illness to do your energy mapping; don't wait until you feel better.

Psychological repair: Weakened psychological, social, or emotional boundaries increase your susceptibility to psychic information and can attract disturbing or inaccurate sources. If the psychic information is providing you with negative insights, work with a therapist or a spiritual counselor. Never reinforce your agitated assumptions about the world.

Closeness: The more intimate you are with someone, dead or alive, the greater is your chance of communicating psychically with them or others. The heart is ultimately about relationships. Invoke relationships with those you trust, whether they are on this or the other side of physical reality, and ask for help.

Near Death Experience (NDE) or high spiritual attainment: Individuals who have been clinically dead and returned to life test as significantly more psychic than non-NDEers, as they are called. The two types of individuals are revealed to be biochemically different, according to brain research. If you've had an NDE, use the gifts that were awakened at that time. If you have shamanic tendencies, journey through your heart into your possible death and ask what you can do to avert a tragedy stemming from your heart condition. If this advice is medically sound, follow it.

Previous psychic experiences: Research also suggests that once you or a family member has had a psychic experience you are more likely to have another one. Comb your memories and family records. Are there any patterns? Follow the path that came before for your own healing purposes.

With your psychic gifts attuned, you are ready to energy map and shift heal on any of the pathways. The following insert shows you how to energy map. It outlines energy information you'll need to know, followed by healing techniques usable on any of the pathways.

Pathway Ideas and Techniques

This insert provides information that is useful to all pathways, as well as diagnostic and healing techniques you can use for energy mapping on every pathway. Let it serve as a reference for you as you work with energy mapping. It covers the following basics:

- Chakra Diagnosis and Healing, page 116
- Other Energy Bodies Vital to Pathway Healing, page 133
- Your Energy Fields, page 136
- Kundalini: The Magic Energy, page 139
- Entities and Energies: Invisible Help and Harm, page 141
- Energy Absorption Issues, page 148

The first five sections provide background information for energy healing and energy mapping, serving as the basis for your energy work.

Following the section on Energy Absorption Issues are exercises and techniques you can use for energy healing. You can refer to the first five sections of this chapter for background information on the following topics:

Like any task, energy healing is easiest if you are relaxed and serene. Before beginning any energy-based exercise, take a few minutes to clear your mind and calm your body. First, clear the space around you. Literally. Eliminate any clutter surrounding the area you are going to work within, and set the lighting for your own comfort. Establish your privacy. Now take a few deep breaths and concentrate on relaxing each part of your body, beginning with your feet. Feel your feet. Imagine they are planted in the ground, anchored securely within the earth. Clench and then release each major muscle group in your body, toe to head, and with a final big breath, ask the Divine to assign guides to attend you. As you open yourself to your intuition, remember that you have been intuitive throughout your life. Now you can begin to work energetically.

Chakra Diagnosis and Healing

There are many different reactions to energy work. Many people feel tingling or sensations of hot or cold. This means you are opening, receiving, or releasing energies. You might experience various feelings, memory flashbacks, strange thoughts, dream-like awareness, or other sensations. Often a backlog of emotions, memories, and thoughts flood out when we open the doors of our chakras. You might feel suddenly afraid or judgmental of the task at hand. This commonly occurs when someone becomes close to an issue or a memory that is frightening but important. Or you might feel nothing at all.

If nothing happens in the moment, observe your feelings, dreams, and thoughts over the next few days. Chances are, you'll experience some changes. Chakras are physical organs, and the body often releases or attracts energy gradually. Some people experience a "healing crisis" within ten days of an energy session. Unblocked emotions, long-standing issues, repressed beliefs, and crusty judgments, when invited forth, can sometimes create the sense of a physical or an emotional catastrophe. If you're patient with the process, you'll soon clear your blockages and experience relief and healing.

Vibrational Considerations

Before you work with vibrational healing, consult a medical professional to determine the exact cause of physical problems and disease. Only then should you consider using vibration to change speed, spin, form, or direction for healing.

Many considerations arise when working with the chakras vibrationally, most relating to the properties of energy explored in chapter 2. It is important to differentiate a chakra's front and back, as well as its inner and outer wheels.

Each in-body chakra begins in the center of the spine. From this center point, the chakra generates a vortex in the front and back of the body, forming a chakra front and a chakra back, as discussed in chapter 4. Chakras eight through twelve are not anchored in the physical body, but they still have a front and back that spin energies which affect the front and back of your body and energy system.

It's easy to distinguish the front from the back of an in-body chakra. The front of a chakra spins in front of your body, and the back emanates in back of your body. Determining the front or back of an out-of-body chakra is just as simple. The front generates energies that affect the front of your body and the front of your in-body chakras, while the back affects the back of your body and the back of your in-body chakras.

There are several ways to find the front and back of your chakras, as well as the inner and outer wheels. Psychically, you can apply your intuition to see the chakras in your mind's eye, sense the operation of your chakras and their separate parts, or listen for tones. A chakra's front and outer wheel will be a little higher pitched than the back and inner wheel counterparts, as the former generates energies that are less dense. Physically, you can work with a pendulum as described in Chakra Work with Shape, Spin, and Speed, later in this insert. Be aware that it's much more difficult to use a pendulum to find the inner and outer wheel.

Following is a brief reference to help you work with the different structures of an individual chakra.

Front and back: Your twelve major chakras each have a front and a back. In general, the front processes your conscious and daily needs; the back processes your unconscious and primal programs.

Left and right: The left side of your body and your chakras process information stereotypically considered feminine—feelings, the unconscious, challenges that concern receiving, and spirituality. The right side of your body and your chakras deal with stereotypically masculine energies—those concerning your everyday life and accomplishments, and issues about giving, conquering, and action.

Infrastructure: Chakras each have an inner and an outer wheel. Both wheels should be spinning in rhythm with each other. The inner wheel regulates the unconscious energies controlled by that particular chakra and can connect you to various planes and zones of existence, other worlds, and other dimensions. The outer wheel is your energetic contact between these other realities and the external physical world. The outer wheel is primarily affected by your here and now, your conscious life and thoughts.

Shape: There are two aspects to shape: spin and form.

- *Spin:* Chakras ideally maintain even spins in both the internal and the external wheels. Both wheels usually move clockwise, pulling necessary energy from various planes and worlds to enable a healthy life. Reverse or counterclockwise spins sometimes indicate a release of toxins. A continual reverse spin anywhere but in the inner wheel of the eighth chakra, or in some of the spaces of the eighth auric band, indicates disease and a loss of life energy.

- *Form:* Form references the various geometric and other contours in which energy can appear, as well as the types of forms that can affect energy. A diseased heart or artery, for instance, has abnormal form. The chakras affected by heart disease will also possess abnormal forms.

A circular, evenly spinning chakra is healthy and functioning normally.

Speed: In general, the lower the chakra, the more slowly it should be moving. When wheels within a certain chakra are moving at contrary speeds, out of rhythm with each other, or out of rhythm with the other chakras, you must evaluate these wheels for bad programming or disease.

Direction: Sometimes a chakra is off-balance and its fulcrum or outsides point off-center. You want a chakra to be centered and emanating even, circular waves. To do so, program a goal directly into a chakra and allow the resulting direction to send and draw energies supportive of your ends.

Color: Psychically, each chakra appears as a certain color. Color is one measure of vibration and also of information. The section called Chakra Diagnosis by Color in this insert diagrams the healthy colors for each chakra. You will need to know these colors to evaluate which chakras are involved in a heart condition and which colors to use in healing.

Symbology: Encoded in each chakra are symbols and numbers holding that chakra in alignment with its core spiritual programming. Unfortunately, the energetics of these symbols can be warped through life's negative influences, poor behavioral choices, or inherited genetic disturbances. You can potentially transform an injured organ, blood vessel, or tissue into a healthier state by energetically transmitting the correct symbol into the damaged site.

Tones: Tones are vibratory, and if you have an auditory gift, you can listen to a chakra to evaluate its health. Chakras causing or affected by heart disease will sound "off tone." *In energy mapping, the reader is listening to the chakras, not the actual heart disease.* You can command changes to the chakra through words, music, tones, or sounds. If you can retune the chakra to the body, you can alter the programming holding the heart problem in place.

Chakra Work with Shape, Spin, and Speed

To determine the shape, spin, or speed of a chakra use a pendulum (a pendulum is any small object on a chain or a string). The subject (or yourself, using someone else as a tester) can either lie down or sit in a chair. It's easiest to evaluate the front and back of chakra spins when someone is lying down.

Hold the pendulum several inches to a foot over a chakra center. You will feel a subtle tug of energy when connecting with the chakra vortex. Keep your hand steady. If linked with the chakra, the pendulum will slowly being to swing. Within a few moments, this swing will take form and pick up speed. When this movement is stabilized, you can evaluate it for function or dysfunction.

A healthy chakra will cause the pendulum to spin in a broad, full circle at a measured speed. The best way to recognize a healthy chakra spin is to find a chakra spin that is off. An unhealthy chakra might have a swing that arcs to the left or right; it might spin really fast or really slow; or it might remain at a standstill or have a large or tight loop. These off-swings are meaningful and can indicate the presence or nature of disease. After seeing a dysfunctional chakra, you can then determine which chakras are healthier.

Techniques for psychically evaluating swing are similar to those provided in the section titled Vibrational Considerations, which appeared earlier in this insert in reference to discerning the front and back and inner and outer wheels of the chakras. In general, a visual sensitive will peer into a chakra for pictures that illustrate a spin. A kinesthetic will sense or feel disturbances. And the verbally gifted will listen for tones that seem distorted or aberrant. If you are verbal, it's best to assess first the general harmonic of the body you are assessing—yours or another person's. To determine your personal harmonic, you can use the exercise, Keying into Your Spiritual Harmonic, mentioned in chapter 7 in this book and described in depth in *Advanced Chakra Healing*. This harmonic can serve as your baseline for evaluating your own chakra health. Tones that are too high-pitched in comparison to the baseline, for instance, can indicate a chakra spin that is too fast. Tones that are too low might reveal a spin that is too slow. To diagnose another person, tune into their personal harmonic and perform the same evaluation you would for your own chakra health.

Evaluating Shape Here are some basic meanings of the general chakra forms as perceived with the pendulum or through psychic vision. To correct situations by manipulating shape, shift energies until the chakra is balanced by creating a new and balanced shape. Use a symbol to hold this new shape; a cross of equal lines always works. I also recommend surrounding this cross with a circle.

- *Round:* This indicates a healthy and balanced chakra.
- *Lacking substance on right (from subject's perspective):* This indicates a chakra that is oriented toward unconscious programming, emotions, and right-brain creativity; it is lacking action and follow-through.

- *Lacking substance on left:* This indicates a chakra that is geared toward conscious behavior and actions and left-brain analysis; it is lacking creativity and intuition.
- *Lacking substance on bottom:* This indicates a chakra that is more spiritual than practical.
- *Lacking substance on top:* This indicates a chakra that is more practical than spiritual.

Evaluating Spin A chakra should hold a solid, even spin. From the point of view of the pendulum holder, a healthy chakra's front spin will cause the pendulum to move clockwise and to the right. A healthy chakra's backswing will appear counterclockwise. To make measurement easier, I describe how to evaluate chakra health from the front only. You will have to reverse the description to analyze the back. Clockwise spins usually indicate health, unless they are moving too quickly. A counterclockwise spin often shows a blockage or a misperception, unless that chakra is temporarily detoxifying. The exception to this guideline is that the eighth chakra's inner wheel will move counterclockwise frequently, because it functions as a central clearinghouse. In general, you want all chakras opened the same amount and spinning at about the same rate. This indicates a balanced system.

Following are the meanings of spins in both the inner and the outer wheels.

- *Round, uniform, and even swing, clockwise:* The chakra is healthy and functioning.
- *Round, uniform, and even swing, counterclockwise:* The chakra is attempting to create health or balance by processing or clearing negative energy.
- *Nonuniform or uneven swing, counterclockwise:* The chakra is blocked and unable to clear itself.
- *Elliptical or straight line in a vertical direction:* The chakra has well-developed but impractical spiritual views, has a closed to real-life perspective, or is unwilling to take action.

- *Elliptical or straight line in a horizontal direction:* The chakra is practical but lacking a spiritual perspective, or closed to divine assistance.
- *Elliptical or straight line, swinging to the right (of the subject):* The chakra is oriented toward action and daily activities but lacks the emotional or spiritual perspective.
- *Elliptical or straight line, swinging to the left (of the subject):* The chakra is oriented toward inspirational, feminine, or intuitive influences but lacks practical, grounding action.
- *Not moving or nearly still:* This indicates a closed chakra. This is a good place to look for a block or cause of a presenting issue.
- *Large swing:* This means the chakra is very open, healthy, and functioning. If the swing is too large and imbalanced in comparison to other chakras, it means the chakra is overstrained and overfunctioning. Determine which chakra this one is compensating for.
- *Small swing:* The chakra is underfunctioning; it must be cleared and opened.

Evaluating Speed The lower the chakra, the slower both chakra wheels should be moving. The inner wheel usually moves at exactly twice the speed of the outer wheel and, except for the eighth chakra, in the same direction. Here are further diagnostic tips.

- *Wheel too slow:* This indicates damage from previous overuse, exhaustion, fatigue, blocks, strongholds, and probably repressed memories or feelings.
- *Wheel too fast:* This indicates current overuse; overstrain; acting to compensate for a weaker chakra or chakra wheel; or a desire to escape certain life events, people, feelings, or issues. It may also be an attempt to release negative energy.
- *Outer wheel fast, inner wheel slow:* This indicates a lack of spiritual, emotional, intuitive, or creative drive or

perspective; underdeveloped beliefs, feelings, or spiritual sense; or an overconcern with physical appearance.

- *Outer wheel slow, inner wheel fast:* This indicates a lack of ability to take action; lack of commitment to follow through, physical drive, or energy; overconcern with spiritual or psychic matters; a fear of moving into the world; or exhaustion in the physical body.

- *Wheels out of synch:* This indicates that inner beliefs and needs don't match with outer reality or action.

Healing Infrastructure with Shape, Spin, and Speed

Here's a list of five basic methods for vibration healing, followed by details you can use as examples for practical application.

- *Infuse with color.* Removing discoloration and permeating the chakra with the correct color can change its shape, spin, or speed.

- *Use symbols.* In the center of each chakra is a symbol representing the fundamental program of the chakra. You can remove negative symbols, repair injured yet accurate symbols, or insert supportive symbols.

- *Use toning.* Tones can eliminate a problem or instill a solution.

- *Examine power levels on the elemental pathway.* Power levels are dualistic energies that trap us into thinking we can't escape, such as perceiving ourselves as a victim or a perpetrator. For more information, see *Advanced Chakra Healing* and Your Energy Fields, later in this chapter.

- *Assess beliefs, feelings, and strongholds.* Dysfunctional beliefs, repressed feelings, and others' feelings form patterns that keep us ill or stuck. Refer to Chakras and Affiliated Heart Conditions in chapter 4 for more information about the links between specific patterns and related chakras.

Chakra Diagnosis by Color

You can diagnose disease or dysfunction using the colors you would expect to see in each chakra when healthy, as shown in the following table.

Chakra	Color	Meaning of Color
One	Red	Passion
Two	Orange	Feelings and creativity
Three	Yellow	Wisdom and power
Four	Green	Healing
Five	Blue	Communication and guidance
Six	Purple	Vision
Seven	White	Spirituality
Eight	Black	Karma: the effect of the past
Nine	Gold	Soul purpose and unity with others
Ten	Earth tones	Relationship to the environment
Eleven	Pink	Transmutation (of negative to positive and vice versa)
Twelve	Clear	Link human with Divine

Harmful Coloration When colors inside the chakra or body are off, you can use this information to identify what is causing the problem. Here are the meanings of various altered colors.

Imbalanced Colors	Meaning of Imbalanced Colors
Added red tones	Overstimulates passion, anger, ego, or survival fears.
Added orange tones	Creates more emotionalism or hyperactivity.
Added yellow tones	Overemphasizes mental ideas or beliefs that create falsehoods or judgments.
Added green tones	Overstimulates a drive for relationships, codependency, and a

	perceived need to heal what doesn't need healing.
Added pink tones	Can create a sense of love where it doesn't exist.
Added blue tones	Causes a perceived need to obtain more and more guidance or to overexplain oneself.
Added purple tones	Causes compulsive planning and difficulties in seeing or sorting out choices.
Added white tones	Overstimulates a sense of spirituality and deemphasizes the need for power and action.
Added black tones	Imbalances spiritual energies with an emphasis on power; can cause powerlessness, emotionalism, or greed.
Added gold tones	Causes excessive idealism and a resulting loss of hope.
Added silver tones	Creates susceptibility to psychic sources.
Added brown tones	Results in confusion, hyperpracticality, and mundane obsessions.
Added gray tones	Shadows or covers an issue, causing a lack of clarity.
Neutralizing	Erasing intensity creates emptiness and powerlessness.
Imposing	Forcing a color over someone else's, thus achieving control over the other person. This is also called creating an "overlay."
Blotching	Creates inconsistency, making it hard for a victim to rely on him- or herself.

Missing Colors and the Missing Self If you perceive empty spaces where there ought to be color or shape, some aspect of the self is probably fragmented and held either in another aspect of the self or elsewhere. *Possession* occurs when an aspect of something else or some external energy lies within your own energy field. *Recession* involves subjugation of an aspect of self in another entity. An exercise for dealing with these issues called Entities and Energies: Invisible Help and Harm appears later in this insert.

Coloring Your Healing Each color listed represents a different type of energy. Adding these colors to a chakra produces the intended effect. You can add colors psychically by picturing the desired hue and infusing it into the depleted area, by sensing the needed color in the weak area, or by imagining a tone that invokes the required color and humming it in your mind. You can also add the missing color to your wardrobe, household, or office.

- Red: Life energy
- Orange: Creativity and feelings
- Yellow: Intellect
- Green: Healing
- Pink/Rose: Love
- Blue: Communication
- Purple: Vision, clarification of choices, and decisions made
- White: Divine will, spiritual destiny
- Black: Power for movement, force behind change
- Gold: Harmony
- Silver: Transference of energy from one place to another
- Brown: Practicality and grounding

Healing with Symbology: Geometric and Number Symbols

To conduct symbol diagnosis and healing, examine the center of the chakra to see which symbol is determining the current state of disrepair. An off-symbol will look twisted, skewed, or misshapen in some way that alters the symbol from wholeness (hence I use the term "altered" to describe these symbols in the following chart). Then consult the spirit-enhancing symbols lists to identify which symbol to replace it with.

Geometric Symbols

Harmful

- Altered Circle: Breaks positive relationships or creates harmful ones
- Altered Square: Is used to overthrow or topple systems
- Altered Rectangle: Imprisons or exposes to danger
- Altered Triangle: Creates illness, disease, imbalance, and death
- Altered Spiral: Forces abrupt endings, cessation of cycles or rhythms
- Altered Five-Pointed Star: Stifles, contains, suffocates
- Altered Six-Pointed Star: Enforces being stuck, despair, and depression
- Altered Cross: Accentuates ego or causes extreme dejection
- X: Is evil or anticonsciousness

Spirit-Enhancing

- Circle: Wholeness
- Square: Foundation
- Rectangle: Protection
- Triangle: Preservation and immortality
- Spiral: Creation and cycles
- Five-Pointed Star: Alchemy and movement
- Six-Pointed Star: Resurrection
- Cross: Human-Divine connection and spiritual protection

Number Symbols Numerical symbols can actually be psychically perceived as numbers that appear in the chakras. Sometimes a kinesthetic person will sense or "just know" a number, while a verbal sensitive will hear a sequence of tones that add up to a number. Whereas spirit-enhancing numbers appear, look, or sound complete, altered numbers appear broken or distorted, feel "off," or sound cut off or out of beat.

Harmful Numeric Symbols

- Altered 1: Prevents you from reaching a conclusion
- Altered 2: Forces unhealthy liaisons; keeps victims stuck on the powerless side of power levels
- Altered 3: Causes chaos
- Altered 4: Imprisons or creates craziness
- Altered 5: Creates trickery or delusion
- Altered 6: Causes confusion and disorder, convincing the victim to choose evil; this is the number of the lie
- Altered 7: Establishes doubt about the Creator's very existence
- Altered 8: Stifles learning and forces the recycling of harmful patterns
- Altered 9: Instills terror and fear about change
- Altered 10: Prevents new beginnings and seeks to make victims continue the old ways
- Altered 11: Obliterates self-esteem and seeks to keep victims from accepting their humanity
- Altered 12: Disavows forgiveness and casts shadows over human goodness

Spirit-Enhancing Number Symbols

- 1: Beginnings; represents the highest form, the Creator
- 2: Pairing and duality; reflects that everything in the material universe is made of opposites, which are the same; a two splits unity but also holds two ones in unity
- 3: The number of creation, which lies between and emanates from a beginning and an ending
- 4: Foundation and stability; the number of complete balance—consider the four-legged stool

- 5: Direction setting; space for making decisions; represents the human figure, able to go in every direction at once or to travel at will
- 6: Choices; the presence of light and dark, good and evil, and gifts of love, as offered through free will
- 7: Spiritual principles; the Divine; the number of love and action that produces grace; key number of the third dimension
- 8: Infinity; recurring patterns and karma; path of recycling; the number of knowledge
- 9: Change; elimination of what was; ending of cycles of the number symbol eight; as the highest single-digit number, nine can erase error and evil and bring us to a new beginning
- 10: New life; release of the old and acceptance of the new; the number of physical matter
- 11: Acceptance of what has been and what will be; release of personal mythology; opening to divine powers
- 12: Mastery over human drama; acceptance of being fully human and seeing the power in it; mystery of the human as divine

Number and Geometric Combinations

Certain geometric symbols derive extra power from their connection with a particular number. For example:

- 1 with a dot or circle: Highlights correct perception
- 2 with a horizontal line: Strengthens partnerships
- 3 with a triangle: Invites creativity
- 4 with a cross that has arms of equal length; also an equilateral triangle: Fixes support
- 5 with a pentagon; also a pentagram: Shows ultimate truth
- 6 with an equilateral hexagram: Reveals correct choices
- 7 with an equilateral septangle; also a rainbow: Prompts miracles

- 8 with an equilateral octagon: Shifts patterns positively
- 9 with three equilateral triangles: Eases change
- 10 with a circle and a cross of eight arms; also a square with a circle in the middle: Brings needed beginnings
- 11 with parallel lines: Opens mastery
- 12 with a corona: Calls divinity

Tone Diagnosis and Healing

All musical notes hold a vibration, and each creates a different result. The human body is attuned to the A note, as explained in my book, *Advanced Chakra Healing*. This means all of the body's physical and energetic systems will balance with A from the core of a chakra outward, especially if the person's heritage is Western. Eastern cultures resonate to a variety of other notes, tending toward chords that are more flat (or sharp), atonal, or chromatic. However, I believe that all life is sensitive to the basic note of A.

Tones can heal, and they also can harm. Off-tones throw your body out of balance. Correct tones blend with your core harmonic and keep you strong. Listen for tones in order to diagnose disease and to check which tones will enable healing.

Here are the meanings of the basic tonal vibrations.

Whole Notes

Note	Attunes to	Role of the Note
A	Spirit	Attunes human to divine nature, your human self to your spiritual self
B	Mind	Attunes your Lower and Middle Mind to the Higher Mind
C	Feelings	Attunes your human feelings to spiritual feelings
D	Body	Attunes your physical body, condition, or material needs to your spiritual body, gifts, or manifesting abilities
E	Love	Attunes whatever is out of love to unconditional divine love

F	Miracles	Attunes any aspect of your being to the spiritual forces needed at that particular time, breaking through duality into the miraculous
G	Grace	Delivers grace, which is divine love and divine power, to the situation at hand

Sharps and Flats: Sharps bring the spiritual into material reality. An F sharp, for instance, activates that part of your internal spirit that links you with the force you now require. Flats allow release. A G flat, for instance, which is the same tone as an F sharp, pushes out any negative or evil forces preventing your spiritual destiny. The difference between working with a sharp and a flat is intention. If you desire to eliminate something, think flat; to attract something, think sharp.

Core Tones: Many esoteric groups, such as the Masonic, New Age, Quabbalistic, and other spiritual traditions, work with a C-based system of musical scales. I point out that there are two versions of the scales. The first is octave-based, in which notes are repeated in eighths. The second version of scales counts in fifths; this is the model that I believe underlies the Primary Grid (a system of spiritual truths that are the foundation for reality), and the divine pathway. I start fifths with an A, then merge the system of octaves into it for healing.

Basic Chakra Tones

Chakra	My Theory	Esoteric Theory
First Chakra	A	C
Second Chakra	B	D
Third Chakra	C	E
Fourth Chakra	D	F
Fifth Chakra	E	G
Sixth Chakra	F	A
Seventh Chakra	G	B

Eighth Chakra	A	C
Ninth Chakra	B	D
Tenth Chakra	C	E
Eleventh Chakra	D	F

The twelfth chakra does not hold one single tone. Because it is representative of collective human traits and is a conglomerate of many secondary chakras, the twelfth can resonate with any tone. You can attune all chakras by sounding a selected tone through the twelfth chakra, which will both physically and psychically transfer the tone to the other chakras.

A more personalized way to determine tonal healing is to establish your own harmonic. See chapter 7, Shift Healing on the Power Pathway, and conduct the exercise Keying into Your Spiritual Harmonic.

Other Energy Bodies Vital to Pathway Healing

Dozens of energy bodies exist. Each pathway has energy bodies unique to itself; a few of these are briefly described in the chapters about each pathway. For a full discussion, you can study my book, *Advanced Chakra Healing*. The auric field, energy egg, and etheric mirror, however, interconnect all the pathways, and it is essential that you be aware of them.

Your Auric Field

While your chakras operate the "you inside of you," your auric field regulates the "you outside of you." There are twelve basic bands in your auric field, just as there are twelve chakras. These two sets of organs are paired together. The first chakra, for instance, is partnered with the first band of the auric field, and so on. Because of this partnership, changes you make through your chakras are automatically translated into your auric field, and vice versa.

The auric field is important for setting boundaries that protect you and screen information. Information has to pass through the parameters of your field in order to connect with your chakras and therefore your body. Communiqués sent from your chakras must pass through the screen of your aura to be delivered into the world. In regard to heart disease, it's important to establish the correct relationship between these two energy bodies. The focus chakra and auric band for heart conditions is usually the fourth, although there are many exceptions. Many diabetics, for instance, develop heart disease when their illness reaches a critical point. The origin of a diabetic-induced heart problem is the third chakra and auric band rather than the fourth, because the third chakra houses the pancreas.

When healing on the four pathways, it's vital to make sure you translate a healing between the partnered chakra and auric band. Let's say you reprogram a chakra for health but haven't yet transferred the energy to the related auric band. It will be difficult to attract the type of support or assistance that you need to gain optimal help. Perhaps you've just had surgery and the ensuing trauma wounds both your auric field and your physical tissues. You must repair the auric field to keep infectious diseases and others' feelings from entering the body and causing more problems. If you can then transfer the auric band repair into the chakra, your internal tissue will mend more quickly. Always coordinate your chakra healing with equivalent healing in the corresponding auric band.

Your Energy Egg

The *energy egg* is an electromagnetic body that penetrates and surrounds your twelve chakras and auric bands. It creates the outer rim of your human energy system, psychically appearing as a pulsating, three-layer field of incandescent energies. Working with the energy egg for healing helps achieve several goals. Through the energy egg, you can:

- Clear the programs or beliefs held in the subconscious and unconscious that might be causing illness and distress
- Connect your higher consciousness to your everyday consciousness, so that you can attract your greatest desires
- Diagnose and then release the negative information and energies causing your illness
- Attract the spiritual energies or "waves" that create real and permanent changes in health and happiness

To work with your energy egg, you must understand the structure of this energy body and how it works with your chakras and auric bands in relationship to your programming.

The Structure of Your Energy Egg   There are three layers to an energy egg. You can connect to any of these layers at will through your pineal gland, but you will most likely link only with the innermost layer unless you have achieved a relatively high state of consciousness.

This *first layer of the energy egg* relays information-energy between your body and inner psyche and the world at large. This first layer is responsible for alerting the world about the messages of your subconscious and for attracting the needs programmed into your brain. Deep psychological, emotional, or otherwise challenging issues are observable in this layer; these will limit your ability to allow energies from the other two layers into your physical self. This layer can be contacted through the pineal gland and also through the twelfth auric band and chakra, the latter of which connects into thirty-two secondary points of energy in your body.

The *second layer of the energy egg* looks psychically like a thin line of energy that intersperses black energies and white energies. This layer attracts that which you imagine within your unconscious. You could call it the layer of wish making and dreaming. If your programming is warped, you will access energies that deter you from your destiny, or you will form fantasies that are unrealistic. If your use of the second layer is healthy, your twelfth chakra and auric band enable the manifestation of desires into your everyday life.

The *third layer of the energy egg* is an incandescent, shimmering body of energy that interconnects the outer rim of the twelfth chakra and auric band and the spiritual realms that lay beyond the human self. This layer attracts only that which fits your highest spiritual needs and purposes; it is therefore connected to what you could call your highest consciousness. This layer can actually call energies into your life that don't yet exist on this planet but which will benefit you and other people. The possibility for producing physical and emotional miracles lies in working with this layer.

The Etheric Mirror

The *etheric mirror* copies your etheric body, which is comprised of the tenth auric band and the first auric band. The etheric body doubles your physical body; though both can be damaged by life experiences and, over time, these two energy bodies become different from each other. The etheric mirror, on the other hand, holds the correct and perfect codes for your physical and energetic body. Through it, you access accurate DNA patterns and use intention, vibrational methods, or various techniques according to pathway to translate these energies directly into the body.

I also call this the Christ body, as the etheric mirror has seemingly magical healing powers. Using the term *Christ* refers to the ancient mystical principle of the human and the divine being interconnected. We each have a Christ nature and the potential for being fully human and divine simultaneously.

Your Energy Fields

Several energy fields are critical to the healing process.

Etheric fields surround every quantum, cell, organ, and living being, as well as many inanimate energies. Etheric materials usually vibrate at octave levels above their corresponding physical cousins. They can generate information that is slower or faster than the speed of light, and they often "catch" information that can cause disease before the physical body incorporates this information. Energies that can lead to heart disease are often first received and held in the etheric field. The etheric field can protect the internal body from stressors only for a limited time, however.

If suddenly overloaded, the etheric field might completely or partially collapse, dumping distorted vibrations into the body, hence the appearance of "overnight" or sudden heart problems. This situation frequently occurs after severe trauma or strain, such as loss of an important relationship, death of someone close, or a car accident. Most of life's stresses are chronic, such as the worrying over a thirty-year mortgage. Bodily tissue then usually mirrors the eventual erosion of the etheric walls around the weakest or most related parts of the system. Relationship concerns corrode both the etheric boundaries and the physical tissues of the heart or relationship chakra. Financial challenges compromise the first-chakra etheric walls and the related organs, such as the adrenals. Stressed adrenals increase the presence of cortisol and other hormones that can eventually lead to heart problems. Each chakra is susceptible in its own way to stresses that can cause heart problems. You can often read the material of the etheric mirror to determine whether an etheric field, energy body, or part of your physical body is uniform with its ideal.

The most basic field is your body's *electromagnetic field.* Electricity conducted through a conduit generates a magnetic field— hence the term *electromagnetic field.* Every part of your body vibrates electrically and therefore produces a magnetic field. The heart, brain, and central nervous system are the three most vital physical systems of your internal electrical system. The heart generates thousands of times more electrical energy than does your brain (the master of the central nervous system, which includes your spine). These three organs or systems interact, sending and receiving information from the external environment into your internal environment, and vice versa. As well, every single cell pulses with electrical information, which serves as a conduit for passing information. Through your electrical system, all cells are able to "reach through" the physical walls of the body and receive direct messages from the world outside of the body. The tiniest atom within a cell nucleus can speak to the stars because information can vibrate everywhere, all at once.

The auric field is really a vibrating set of magnetic fields (which hold some electrical properties) both around and, to an extent, within your physical body. This means the energies that affect and are generated by your auric field will vibrate throughout every part of your body.

A lack of vitality in your magnetic field will greatly weaken the affected auric band, as well as your entire auric field, making you more susceptible to disease. Too much electrical energy in your auric field, in comparison with your magnetic field, and you'll attract negative energies—such as others' emotions or issues—into your body. As you can imagine, the health of your heart, as the major electrical organ in the body, is highly affected by issues of electromagnetism.

Morphogenetic fields convey information from one person or one group to another. There are morphogenetic fields connecting all animals, the various species, all humans, and people within a country or members of a family. Heart problems, or the vibrations causing them, can be shared through various morphogenetic fields; this accounts in part for tendencies toward certain heart diseases specific to ethnic or family types.

The *Vivaxis* is a word coined by naturopath Judy Jacka to describe the various networks of fields that operate through and around the planetary globe. Some of these energetic fields connect the earth to other planets and planes; others link us to the electromagnetic fields on this planet. Many heart problems are caused or impacted by geopathic stress (a concept introduced in chapter 2). Fields generated from microwaves, radio stations, power lines, nuclear power plants, and more cause vibrational damage to our own etheric fields and warp the heart's electrical function. Even the electrical fields from mercury dental implants can negatively impact our electrical field and create heart abnormalities!

The fields listed here, plus others, are part of what I call the *Secondary Grid*, an interlocking network of energetic lines, fields, and forces that cause duality on this planet and in our bodies. *Duality* is the belief that there are oppositional energies. If someone perceives herself to be a victim all the time, for instance, she will be unlikely to contact the energies that can make her more powerful. In reference to cardiovascular disease, if you believe yourself to be a victim of your heart, it will be difficult for you to see your heart as a victor of love, and therefore as its own source of healing. In contrast, we can also choose to operate on the *Primary Grid*, a star-studded formation of spiritual truths that occupy the divine pathway.

Part of the Secondary Grid is a series of power levels and power fields that relate to the inception of strongholds in your body. *Power levels* are consciousness waves that hold two dualistic notions together. They can capture your thoughts and energies and keep you imprisoned in your mental and emotional strongholds. *Power fields* are a progressive order of energetic fields that stair-step you through the human development process into owning your divinity. A complete outline of power levels and power fields is available in my book, *Advanced Chakra Healing*. I heartily recommend working with power levels and fields if you have heart disease—you can achieve stellar results.

Kundalini: The Magic Energy

Kundalini is an ancient Hindu term for the spiritualizing of the energy system and a process for unfolding your life-force energy; it is extremely important in the healing of heart disease. Heart problems often involve stifled or sometimes overstimulated kundalini. If the kundalini fails to rise through the body, for instance, this red-colored and enflaming energy will remain burning in the adrenals. Enflamed or burned-out adrenals create internal stressors that can lead to heart problems. Kundalini stuck in the liver can stimulate the overproduction of cholesterol. If this blazing energy is trapped in the heart, it creates inflammation, one of the leading proponents of heart problems. Lack of kundalini in the fourth chakra might cause irregular heartbeat (as can too much kundalini). Trace the path of the kundalini and you can often find the source of a heart problem.

The kundalini process unfolds in every pathway except the imagination pathway; when complete, it unifies the Four Pathways system. In its primary stage, kundalini starts on the elemental pathway, in the first chakra for men and the second chakra for women; the kundalini then rises through the remainder of the energy system and comes full circle.

Kundalini energy empowers your entire body in accord with your spirit and can therefore bring your correct harmonic into each and every part of your body.

You can induce your kundalini on three of the pathways using these techniques:

- On the elemental pathway, work with *serpent* or *red kundalini* to clear the body of energetic blockage. Red kundalini is the most primary of kundalini energies; it keeps the body healthy and balanced.

- On the power pathway, use *golden kundalini* from above to spiritualize the red kundalini and access spiritual powers. Golden kundalini is a spiritual energy that enters from above the head. When it merges with the red kundalini, it helps your body achieve the state of health that matches your spiritual nature.

- On the divine pathway, *radiant kundalini* emanates from each and every cell, organ, and aspect of the self upon claiming divine love. Radiant kundalini is unique to itself, though when it generates from inside of you, it joins the red and golden kundalini and therefore completely brings all aspects of your life to your highest physical and spiritual potentials.

- On the imagination pathway there is no energy, so you can't use kundalini there. However, actions on the imagination pathway affect kundalini positively or negatively.

Entities and Energies: Invisible Help and Harm

Invisible entities and energies can help or harm you. The two features to understand are sourcing and interference.

Sourcing

A *source* is an origin of information or energy. *Sourcing* involves tracing a problem or issue back to its original sources, which might be people, experiences, ideas, entities, consciousnesses, or energies that have wrongly informed you.

Heart problems can start with inanimate or animate sources. *Inanimate sources* aren't alive, but most inanimate sources generate fields and share information. Bad fats can be an inanimate source of heart disease. In addition to the obvious physical disturbances created by trans fats, their frequency can disrupt the function of liver and circulatory cells. *Animate sources* are beings with consciousness. They don't have to be alive. A ghost or an angel, for instance, is an animate source. Animate sources do, of course, include people. *Helpful sources* encourage the internalizing of your personal spirit in your body, whereas *harmful sources* discourage this internalization.

When working with heart disease, we almost always have to identify a source for the cause. Don't assume the heart organ is the origin of all heart issues. Problems in other organs, and therefore chakras, can cause the initial disturbance. Diseased kidneys, which are affected by the first, second, or third chakra, affect the body's cell salts and therefore circulation. The kidneys are known esoterically as the storage of childhood fears and ancestral issues. We might have energies from childhood that have resulted in kidney problems and, subsequently, heart problems. Uncovering the root of a heart problem might involve many forms of alternative work, including regression, hypnotherapy, dream work, or simply memory recall to find out whether (and if so, where) we have taken on disruptive energies from an external source.

Sources can be positive and life enhancing, as well as harmful or destructive. All aspects of yourself are available to help with healing and manifesting, and there are countless divine-oriented sources to assist you in your healing endeavors. In the individual chapters on the pathways, I have listed the sources that are likely to be most helpful on each pathway. Among the sources listed are natural forces, natural spirits, nature spirits, elemental beings, beings of the stars, beings of earth, natural objects, angels, masters, avatars, ascended masters, saints, spirit guides, extraterrestrials, allies, forms and powers, and ancestors.

Interference

Interference occurs when an internal or external source of energy interrupts your natural harmonic in a harmful way. Some sources will disturb your natural harmonic to benefit you; for example, to open up a new life choice or to make you aware of potential danger. I use the term *interference* to describe interruptive negative sources, such as those that cause tragedy, trauma, and disease.

There are many types of interference, and all can be involved in establishing conditions that initiate heart problems. The major types are entity based, or consciousness based, aspects of the self or energetic contracts.

Interference can directly cause the conditions for heart problems or attach someone to energies that can create heart disease. Congenital heart defects, for instance, are begun in utero.

Although the obvious physical cause is genetic, on the Four Pathways approach, we ask, "What stimulated the genetic material to form a heart problem?" Perhaps an interfering ancestor attached an energetic contract to serve its own purposes, thus activating an abnormal gene. Invading or interfering information from all sources, including one's own soul, can be programmed into the body through physical or energetic genetics. *Energy genetics* is the sharing of information that codes your energy system first and your physical system and genetics second.

Following are lists of the various types of interfering energies that might cause, support, or enhance cardiovascular disease. More detailed descriptions are provided in my book *Advanced Chakra Healing*.

- *Entity-based interference* involves an *entity*, or a being, with its own unique spirit and a soul. Through its soul, an entity traverses time and space to gather experiences. Entities most likely to initiate heart conditions include ancestors, harmful souls, hauntings (which I'll describe shortly), and living people who project an aspect of themselves into or around you.

- *Sorcery* is interference from an energy, an entity, or a consciousness that seeks to control its subject through manipulation.

- *Consciousness-based interference* can be group energy, such as group consciousness, or powerful ideas that brainwash people into thinking or acting a certain way. These can actually be supported by a consciousness fear, or a *group consciousness*, a collection of thoughts that seek to influence the thoughts of others. If we buy into the group fear of intimacy, for instance, we will be afraid to give and receive love. This fear locks into our bodies in our heart organ, thus creating vibration distortions that throw off the heart muscle and create physical strain, such as problems with oxygenation, rhythm, or blood cleansing.

Aspects of the Self

The source of a heart condition often lies no farther than the mirror. There are many, many aspects of the self to consider when sourcing heart problems, but the basic ones are these:

- Your spirit, which is the immutable and eternal aspect of the self. Your spirit is often the medic for heart problems, but it can sometimes allow the condition for higher learning, usually around the topic of unconditional love.

- Your soul, which carries you through time and through experience, gaining wisdom and wounds along the way. The soul often supports heart problems because it fears unconditional love. Heart disease is a paradoxical way to learn how to open the heart to love. It can also reinforce love avoidance.

- Your mind, which regulates your thinking and beliefs. Few beliefs invite love, because love involves intimacy and being vulnerable to being wounded.

- Your heart, which connects all aspects of yourself through love. Our major heart fear is that we are unlovable. A closed heart isn't susceptible to having this fear confirmed.

- Your body, which experiences all that life has to offer in order to achieve your spiritual purpose. All organs and their related chakras have individual requirements for healthy functioning. Disturbances in any of these areas can affect the physical and energetic heart.

Within the self are other aspects that can inadvertently create a heart condition. Examples include the personality; the ego; inner children and the innocent child; the God self, primal self, and master self; and the High, Middle, and Low Heart, Mind, and Self. Sometimes one of these aspects desires a heart condition! For instance, an abused inner child might remain energetically stuck within the heart tissue as a way of avoiding his or her abusers. When the abuser comes near, the child strikes out, causing an electrical disturbance that might actually alter the heart's rhythm.

The soul is frequently responsible for heart conditions because it carries issues from lifetime to lifetime. There are several parts to the soul, including soul fragments—individual and often independently operating parts of the soul. A soul might fragment due to trauma and be therefore susceptible to (1) disease; (2) possession, the act of being taken over by another entity or energy; or (3) recession, which involves being stuck in an aspect of something or someone else. Possession and recession can occur with or through any aspect of the self. A possessive being can throw off the heart's rhythm or disturb the healthy function of an organ; missing a recessed aspect of self makes you vulnerable to others' issues, feelings, and energies, as well as physical invaders like bacteria.

Energetic Contracts

Energy contracts are agreements made between two or more entities or energies that create a negative energy exchange. Here are some of the many types of energy contracts that might underlie heart disease.

- A *binding* is an energy force that puts one person or entity in charge of another.
- A *curse* is a binding that holds a group of people in bondage. For instance, a family can be cursed with conditions that cause anemia, high cholesterol, or weakened blood vessels.
- A *miasm* is the product of a familial curse and an attempt to keep everyone similar within a family system. It fixes disease patterns in the etheric energy and so operates like an energetic genetic pattern, predisposing all members of a family, or certain types of family members, to a particular disease or condition.
- A *haunting* is a ghost or an entity that forces the living into certain behaviors. A haunting can't cause heart disease, but

it can nag you into negative behaviors—such as smoking, eating sugar, or drinking alcohol—that can lead to heart problems. A haunting can also reinforce negative beliefs, such as "I am not lovable," which affect the emotional health of your heart.

- A *spell* is a binding held over an individual for control purposes. A spell can distort all or part of your harmonic and cause discord within various cells, which affect their functionality.

- An *energy cord*, a subset of *energy contract*, keeps you connected to another person or group. You can actually pass the programming or patterning for heart problems from one person to another through an energy cord. A *life energy cord* is the most dangerous, because the person on the other end exploits your life energy, which greatly lowers your body's immunity and kundalini. Your heart must receive life energy to keep pumping.

- An *enigma* is a cord that ends in an attachment in your physical body and allows someone else either to drain your life-giving energy or to dump their negative energy into you. Enigmas differ from other types of cords and contracts in that there isn't a two-way flow of energy involved. Someone can simply drain your energy. Enigmas might drain your heart or any other part of the body. A poorly functioning liver won't cleanse your blood correctly, for example, and this can lead to heart problems.

- *Energy markers*, which are similar to enigmas, form counterclockwise spins, usually in symbol form, that drain your vital energy from you. The difference between an energy marker and an enigma is that the loss of energy may or may not involve another person. You might be leaking energy, but this energy isn't necessarily going into something or someone else. This energy might leak into the general atmosphere, and if this energy is negative, it can instruct others to treat you in a negative way.

- *Holds* are often the product of childhood heart conditions and are energetic clamps that keep the child from developing into his or her individual self. These holds might stem from the parents or ancestors, but they are just as likely to be sourced from a religion, culture, group mind, or the child him- or herself. Holds always indicate a personal fear of growing into the person one can become. The internal question is this: "Is it safe to be who I really am?"

- A *codependent contract* is a contract that you make with someone else that ends up doubling back on you. Codependency involves giving to someone else in order to receive what you want from him or her. The end result is inflammation in the areas absorbing another's energies and a lowered immune system from the giving away of your own energy. These are two key factors in the physical development and progression of heart disease. Energetically, the codependent cord forms a figure eight, with the center point located over the original cord site. This center is frequently the heart in the case of heart disease, but not always. Energy transfers throughout the figure eight, which can account for many conditions leading to heart disease.

- Others' energies can cause heart disease, too, throwing your body or parts of it off-key. By internalizing someone else's negative thinking in your throat chakra, for instance, you can disrupt your thyroid. Doctors frequently track heart palpitations to a dysfunctional thyroid. Interference can only be released once you discover your *payoff*—the reason that some aspect of the self allowed the interference.

For more thorough instruction on how to look for and deal with energy contracts, refer to the descriptions of energy contracts and cords in my book *Advanced Chakra Healing.*

Energy Absorption Issues

As I've stressed, energies you pick up from others can cause heart disease in you or create the conditions for it. Others' energies don't resonate within your own system. Intense energies or those absorbed over a long period of time can eventually distort organ function, circulatory health, and even DNA. Internalized energies can also keep your body from responding to a heart crisis. Here are the different types of energies you can absorb and tips on how to recognize a problem.

Feelings

There are five major feeling groups or constellations: anger, sadness, happiness, fear, and disgust. You must deal with your own feelings to heal from heart problems, but you won't get anywhere trying to heal someone else's emotions! There are many ways to know whether you have taken on others' feelings. The easiest determinant is to ask your intuitive self to separate your own feelings from those of others. What doesn't belong to you belongs to someone else. Ask the Divine to clear issues that aren't your own.

Beliefs

There are six primary types of beliefs:

Primary Belief	Negative Aspect	Positive Aspect
Worthiness	I am unworthy	I am worthy
Deserving	I don't deserve	I do deserve
Power	I am powerless	I am powerful
Value	I have no value	I am valuable
Love	I am not loveable	I am loveable
Goodness	I am bad (or evil)	I am good

You can arrive at any of these beliefs on your own. You can also take on others' beliefs and live them out. The key to sorting your own from others' beliefs is to center yourself in your heart and ask to know intuitively your own essential beliefs in regard to an issue. Any ideas or thoughts that don't align with your essential beliefs don't fit for you.

Illnesses and Diseases

To identify when you have taken on another's illness or disease, center in the chakra with the presenting problem. Visual psychics should think of a presenting illness and ask it to form an image. Now ask to see the source of this image. If it's not you, you'll know. Verbal psychics can ask to speak to the illness and demand that it honestly share its source. Kinesthetic psychics might first move into the state of the pure self, then imagine the illness dwelling as a contained energy within the first chakra. They can demand that a personal illness remain within the chakra and that anything not of the pure self be expelled.

Patterns

You've likely absorbed someone else's pattern if one of the following rings true:

- You can't explain certain repetitive actions or behaviors within your own life story.
- No matter how hard you work on breaking a particular pattern, you can't.
- You feel like you are "under a spell," as if compelled into certain repetitive ways of being.
- You keep acting just like Mom or Dad, and you don't want to do so.

In the remainder of this insert, I offer techniques and processes for energy work and energy mapping.

Five Steps for Safe Psychic Use

Here is a five-step process for safely applying your psychic gifts to all energy work. I encourage you to use this process in all your Four Pathways undertakings.

1. *Ground and center. Grounding* involves anchoring your consciousness in a secure and trustworthy substance, such as the earth itself, a place of knowledge, a natural or spiritual force, or a spiritual quality. *Centering* involves locating your fully conscious self where you can access all your gifts and truths. You can center in a part of your body, an energy center, a concept, or a truth.

2. *Establish parameters.* Boundaries keep us inside ourselves and keep what could harm us outside ourselves. There are different forms of boundaries for each pathway. To establish the appropriate parameters for each pathway, use your key actions: intention on the elemental pathway, commanding on the power pathway, imagination on the imagination pathway, and petitioning on the divine pathway.

3. *Achieve the goal.* When energy mapping, you will establish an objective and proceed toward it by following a list of tasks that has been laid out.

4. *Release energies.* In the course of achieving your goal, you may have freed up energies that now must be released from your energy system. In the chapters on the four pathways, there are exercises for eliminating energies that aren't your own.

5. *Center, ground, and reestablish parameters.* Returning to your center is a way of returning to your everyday self. You can then ground in the appropriate energy and set parameters for everyday functioning.

Freeing Yourself from Others' Energies and Interference

Here are different ways to free yourself from energies that might be hampering you.

Reexamine Energy Contracts

Determining the nature of an energetic contract will help you choose the best method for removing it. To decipher a contract, respond to these questions:

- Am I one of the original creators of this contract?
- If I am not an original creator of this contract, how did I come to receive it? Is there something I must do, say, understand, or express to release myself from this contract?
- If I did enter this agreement, when did I do so? For what reason?
- What type of contract is this? An energetic cord? Life energy cord? A binding or an enigma? A codependent contract? If one of the latter, who else is involved in or affected by this agreement?
- What is the nature of the contractual agreement? What am I giving? What am I receiving?
- How is this contract affecting me, the others around me, or the others in the contract?
- What do I need to know to release myself from, to change, or to better use this contract?
- What feelings must I understand or express? What beliefs must I accept? What energy must I release or accept? (On the elemental pathway, ask these questions: What power levels must I free myself from? What power field must be brought to its optimum function?)
- What forgiveness or grace must I allow myself or the others involved?

- Am I now ready for this healing? If not, why not, and when will I be?

There are three main ways of exorcising energy contracts; these methods also work for hauntings. They are different from cord or binding release in that they rely on your power to command and hold intention, rather than a healing process.

- *Rejection.* To reject a contract or interference, you must use 100 percent intention to refuse the contract and repel the energies attached to it. Might is right. If you command with more energy or intelligence than what's used against you, you will win. Request that all concerned receive divine healing from wounds remaining from eliminated contracts.
- *Containment.* You have the divine right to isolate yourself from negative sources. Simply command that the Divine immediately protect you. If you are mightier than your "foe," you can also demand the containment of any energies, forces, or entities that have been plaguing you.
- *Transformation.* By giving the energy of forgiveness, you are sending white light at the energy or entity that is bothering you. This energy offers grace to the interference or contract partners. If they accept the forgiveness, divine love offers healing, and they automatically release you. If they don't, the white light pushes them out of your boundaries and deals with them. Any energy that the other forces have been holding is automatically returned to you when you request transformation for all concerned.

Use the Transpersonal Process

If you think you're dealing with assumed energies, you can conduct this twelve-step, elemental pathway–based healing process:

1. Center yourself in the issue and ask the Divine to separate your own energies from those of others. Ask your own energy to step aside and wait a while. You will communicate with it shortly.

2. Command that energies not your own create an image that can speak and communicate with you.

3. Demand that the energy now present itself in a representation that shows its truest form or nature.

4. Ask why this energy joined with you. What did it want to receive by this action? What did it receive?

5. What did it take from you?

6. Now ask the energy of yourself, currently separated out, what you received from joining with the other energy. What was your payoff? What did you expect to receive?

7. What did you actually receive?

8. Ask yourself what you need to do, own, know, feel, learn, or experience to release the energy that is not your own.

9. Ask the other's energy what it needs to do, own, know, feel, learn, or experience to be willing to leave.

10. Release the energy that is not your own. If it doesn't want to go, ask for divine assistance. This is your right.

11. Repair any damage to your chakric field, then cement it and your auric band back into place. Use healing techniques that conform to your intuitive style. For example, if your style is visual, fill in energy holes with colors or shapes that address apparent problems; if verbal, ask for divine help, command repair on the Power Pathway, or use appropriate tones; if kinesthetic, sense or feel the desired state and make it reality. Ask for divine assistance and for healing now and as you integrate this change.

12. Commit to acting in a whole way for yourself.

Find Your Fragments and Reclaim Yourself

Not only do we implant others' energies but we also give our own energy and parts of ourselves away. The following ten-step process works for recession and cordage to the self.

1. Ground and center.

2. Track the recessed energy to its location. You can look for cords, bindings, filaments, energy lines, and attachments; follow the flow of neutrons; or simply ask to see where the missing self or energies are at this time. If you are verbal, you can attune with your heartbeat and listen for the rhythm of the missing self in the universe.

3. Acknowledge the presence of the Divine in and around you for safety.

4. Psychically look at the situation. Are you caught or trapped? Stuck somewhere else? What aspect of the self is externalized and why? How is your life affected by the lack of this self, energy, or gifts?

5. What needs to occur to integrate this self or energy again? What do you need to know, understand, do, or learn? What does this self or energy need to know, understand, do, or learn?

6. When you are ready for integration, ask the Divine to bring the healing or to release teams of angels and other guardians of the Divine to assist. Allow this self or energy to be fully purified, cleansed, and transformed for integration, and ask that room be made inside of you for it.

7. Ask the Divine to deal with energies that are not your own—whatever or whoever was holding the externalized self—and to completely sever and heal you from any energetic attachments.

8. As you allow integration, ask that you be told anything you must do to support a safe and easy incorporation.

9. Repair any damage to your chakric field, then cement it and your auric band back into place. Using your primary intuitive

gift, use color, shape, or tones to bring the stricken energy body into its proper form. Ask for Divine assistance and for healing now and as you integrate this change.

10. Commit to acting in a whole way for yourself.

Energetically Cleanse with Physical Properties

Repairing after an energetic release can take some time. Here are some elemental pathway–based measures that can speed the process, aid in recovery after possession and integration work, and help you cleanse others' energies on a daily basis.

- *White wash:* Picture the Divine's white energy flooding your body as if through a fountain, flowing from above, through your body, then down through your tenth chakra. Ask that the earth, which will recycle these energies, transmute them.
- *Black tea bath:* Boil five or six black tea bags in one gallon of water over high heat for ten minutes. Remove the tea bags and add only the liquid to your bath. Set the intention of flushing feelings and toxins that are not useful. When done, add colloidal oatmeal to the bath or use baking soda on your skin to restore your skin's pH.
- *Implements:* Select a rock, an amulet, or another tool. With intention, use it to absorb others' energies. Cleanse weekly in the rain, in Epsom salts and water, or through intention.
- *Shaman techniques:* Use candles, incense, drumming, or burning sage to cleanse yourself or your home of others' energies.

Moving through Time for Information and Healing

By moving backward, sideways, and forward in time, you can determine the causes of various problems and find solutions. Here are three basic techniques.

Regressing   Regressions involve looking back into the past, or relinking with a part of you that is stuck in the past, in order to gather data regarding a current problem. You can also potentially use regression to free yourself from the past and to change the past so that the present can be different.

Caution: For serious or frightening issues, I suggest you work with a professional to conduct a regression. Certified hypnotherapists are trained to work with the issues and feelings that arise, as are licensed psychologists trained in Eye Movement Desensitization and Reprocessing (EMDR), a particularly helpful form of regression therapy. For less serious issues, here is a five-step process you can use.

Regression Exercise

1. Prepare. Ground and center. Think of your causal issue. After asking the Divine for protection and guidance, ask which chakra is key to this causal issue. Now open your psychic senses by asking the Divine to open your chakras fully and to allow only loving use of your gifts.

2. Enter. Sense or see the chakra center causal to your issue. There you will spot a door, a mirror, or an opening of some sort. Ask the Divine to guide you through this portal and into the situation that has created your current predicament.

3. Research and clarify. Once in the situation, ask to see, hear, know, and experience everything necessary to obtain the information or healing you need. State that your conscious self will remember all that you are experiencing. Then ask to understand what decisions you (or someone else) made during this time period that still affect you today. Now ask for clarification. Why did you make these decisions? What other choices were available? What did you need to learn? What do you still need to learn?

4. Heal. Ask the Divine to tell you what healing and forgiveness is necessary. Is it appropriate to change the circumstances of that time? How are you to do so? If you are to leave the situation status quo, ask what wisdom will enable you to leave the

past in the past. Now ask the Divine to help you make any necessary changes in the prior time period. Accept the healing energies.

5. Return and infuse. Ask the Divine whether it is appropriate to bring any changes forward so as to affect the present. Is it more helpful simply to make changes in the present, and if so, which ones? Remain in the situation until you feel complete and whole with what happened and who you were at that time. Now request the Divine to return you to the present and to bring with you the learning, energy, wisdom, and information you need to make today a better place. Ask the Divine to help you internalize all appropriate learning or healing through all of your levels in a way that will be safe and easy. Establish any new boundaries for your now-changed self. Ground and center, and return fully to the present. Ask the Divine for additional protection and guidance as you integrate this information and infuse the past into the present.

Projecting

Projecting is a form of shamanic journeying. When journeying, mystics send an aspect of themselves or their consciousness in search of wisdom, data, or healing energies.

Journeying can take you near or far, into the past, present, or future, but it isn't always easy to do without guidance. I use the term *projecting* to describe journeying into only the present time.

On the divine pathway, healing occurs through expansion. Projecting is an elemental pathway–based means of exploring all corners of reality; who knows what or where holds the data or healing you need. Here is a five-step process for using projection for healing purposes.

Projecting Exercise

1. Prepare. Using the steps of grounding, centering, and protecting, ask the Divine to connect you fully with your spirit-self. Breathe deeply and imagine that you are fully invested

in your spirit, which is inside of your body and also able to expand fully around you. Encompass your body in your own spirit, then "feel out to the edges."

2. Travel. Sense the presence of your spirit, which continues to envelop your body, as it swells into the room and then outdoors. Notice that nothing hurts you; everything simply is what it is. Your spirit is inviolate and remains its own pure self no matter what it touches or surrounds. Now think of your causal issue. Simply expand your consciousness as your spirit enters a place or space that contains everything you have yet to learn about this issue. You have now journeyed to exactly where you need to be, without leaving your body behind.

3. Learn. What learning has been awaiting you in this space-time? What wisdom is yours to acknowledge and to grasp? Why is it important to understand this information, in reference to the "you" of the "current time"?

4. Embrace. Fully embrace both this spacetime and the knowledge that you came to learn. Know that you are really embracing yourself.

5. Infuse and return. As quickly as possible, infuse the learning and the spirit-self of the visited spacetime through the energy field connecting the body-based self with the traveling self. As you accept the learning into the here and now, decide to live fully in this body, in this time, with the energies of Truth. Ask the Divine to help you internalize all appropriate learning or healing through all of your levels in a way that will be safe and easy. Establish new boundaries for your now-changed self. Ground and center, and return fully to the present. Ask the Divine for additional protection and guidance as needed, until you are fully integrated.

Futuring

The future is really a net of possibilities that surround your current self. You don't have to "go anywhere" to access the future.

The lines of the future are being drawn around you as you sit and read this book! Here is a five-step process for futuring.

Futuring Exercise

1. Prepare. When futuring, first ground, center, and resonate with your spirit-self. Then attune with the energies of the future that are around you already. You'll see that it's like being surrounded by a grid of Christmas lights! These are magnetic, proton-based timelines that link to possible futures. What do you desire to see? What is your goal? Look at all the twinkling opportunities and times that respond to your question. What is the best path? Ask the Divine to assure you of your choice, as you prepare for "liftoff."

2. Travel. Ask the Divine to show which line your spirit would follow if it weren't affected by adversity or disease. Know that futuring doesn't actually entail any sort of traveling. Instead of sending your consciousness into the future, pull the lighted line as if you are fishing. Reel the line to the front side of your heart and ask to perceive it with True Vision—the vision of your own spirit.

3. Learn. What do you perceive? Ask the Divine to guide you to respond to the images pulled from the future. Are you to learn from it? Own it? Magnetize this potential so it occurs, or do the opposite?

4. Embrace or heal. Can you accept the learning and healing from the future or the future self? If affirmative, assume a position of gratitude for the knowledge or healing received, and allow the future web to shape around you. Embrace the future in the here and now.

5. Infuse and integrate. Close your eyes and connect again with your body. Ground, center, and resonate with the decisions you have made. Ask the Divine to help you continue to integrate your choices safely and with love toward yourself and others.

Healing Feelings

Not all feelings are assumed from others. Here is a high-level spiritual exercise to heal feelings of your own that might fortify an issue.

1. Select an issue or a problem. Accept the discomfort it is causing in your life and in your body. Don't resist.

2. Know that this discomfort does not exist in every aspect of yourself. There are different versions of the same reality. There is a place where you have illness, issues, a problem, or a need, and a space in which your needs are fulfilled in a way that makes the problems unnecessary. If there is discomfort inside of you, there is also a space where there is comfort.

3. Breathe deeply and associate with this state of comfort. A visual psychic may picture the discomfort as a form apart from the body. A kinesthetic intuitive will have to feel the discomfort and move through it until finding a place of clearness in the body. A verbal psychic will command him- or herself to a comfortable space. You can say that you want to be in your "place of purity" or the "state of comfort." If none of these methods works, ask for divine help. You simply want your consciousness placed in the state of comfort.

4. Now the critical element: Feel the feeling connecting you to the discomfort. And I mean feeling as in part of an emotion, not the emotion itself. A discomfort is always energetically composed of a variety of feelings, beliefs, energies, and even entities and forces. This aggregate energy connects with you because at some moment in time you had a feeling about what was going on. Get back to your original feeling.

5. Keep feeling. If another feeling arises, stay with it or consider getting a friend or therapist to help you go to the core feeling.

6. Accept your awareness about the feeling and ask yourself why you had this feeling. This feeling arose historically

because of a perceived need. What was it? What need is this feeling pointing out?

7. Petition to feel the Divine's acceptance of your need. *Look for patterns, strongholds, illnesses, or issues that stem from a need you believe has not been met.* The need has not been met because you judged it, not because the Divine judged it. When we judge a need, we freeze the feeling about the need, then we go about creating distorted ways to get our need met.

8. Petition for the Divine to meet the original need.

9. Know that you can now complete your relationship with the original feeling. This knowledge will open to an even deeper level of truth and eventually give way to a spiritual feeling. The spiritual feeling will generate through the superluminal body, activating the spiritual genetics and changing the conditions in your body. Your spiritual genetics are described in chapter 7. For now, know that they are basically your ideal genetics, as provided by your spirit.

10. Accept the learning. It will change you.

Forgiveness

Forgiveness is a gift to the self. The Greek word for *forgiveness* means to let go or release. It is a way of leaving the past behind to allow you to be free in the present. Which energies are meant to be given to someone else and which are meant to be kept to yourself? Which energies were meant to be kept by someone else and which were meant for you?

Forgiveness Exercise Here is a forgiveness exercise that invites spiritual healing.

1. Invoke the Divine's energy of grace, which is power in love.

2. Center and ask the Divine to help you generate the actual substance of grace outward, from your center to all other aspects of your self.

3. Petition the Divine to grant grace to anything and anyone who has harmed you or continues to affect you negatively. Ask the same for yourself.

4. Offer choices. The conscious direction of grace offers three choices to all individuals, entities, and consciousnesses currently preying on you: to transform, to leave, or to receive consequences. Regardless of what choice another being makes, you can make one that is self-loving and self-respecting, which will involve freeing the others' energies from you. If at first an energy or entity doesn't leave when invited to do so, either contain or rebuke it by handing it over to its higher self or to the Divine.

5. Complete the healing. Invite the Divine to complete the healing by returning your own energies to you, establishing the correct parameters for your renewed integration, and blessing the other people or beings.

Steps to Energy Mapping

You can produce an energy map for each pathway or select one pathway to begin your healing. Generally, the same steps are involved in energy mapping on any of the pathways. I will share an example of energy mapping on the elemental pathway, because it is, paradoxically, the most complicated of the four pathways.

There are two parts to the energy mapping process: diagnosis and healing. Here are the steps:

Part One: Diagnostic Steps

1. Get paper and pen or prepare some other way to remember the information you will be receiving. You will be energy mapping pictorially, drawing or making other notes to record what you learn in these diagnostic steps. Visual psychics can simply sketch what they see. If you receive verbal or tonal information, write down descriptions of what you

hear and in which chakras. The same applies for kinesthetic information; describe the types of feelings you receive in answer to different questions.

2. Ground and center.

3. Establish parameters.

4. Select a starting chakra. Refer to the chart of the various types of heart conditions and their partnered chakras in chapter 4, or trust your intuition to determine your baseline chakra. With heart disease, you can always start with the heart chakra. Access your strongest psychic gift or the gift that's most logical to use in order to energy map.

5. You will now examine the primary disease chakra for diagnostic issues according to your selected pathway. The particular questions you should ask on specific pathways are listed in the chapters about each pathway. Generic issues to examine include the following:

   - Type of charge: negative, positive, or neutral
   - Spin of the chakra or organ involved
   - Spin of the chakra's inner and outer wheels
   - Coloration of the diseased area versus the rest of the chakra
   - Tone of the diseased area versus the rest of the chakra
   - Symbology of the diseased area and symbols in the rest of the chakra
   - Location of interference and connections to other places
   - Connections of the heart to other chakras; for instance, check to see whether there are cords connecting the diseased area to other chakras or energies in the body
   - Connections of the diseased area to other aspects of the self, such as spirit, soul, mind, heart, and body

6. Record your answers on your paper or diagram. After illustrating your responses, examine your findings and go deeper intuitively. Now write the responses you receive when considering each of the following:

- Reason for the heart condition. For instance, with negatively charged heart problems, look for emotional, physical, or psychic causes as well as issues with power; with positively charged heart conditions, look for spiritual beliefs and fears; with neutral heart problems, look for the need for love.

- Onset of the heart condition. When did this heart problem start? You can look to prior existences and prebirth, as well as this lifetime.

- Source of the heart condition. Did the heart problem begin inside of you or with something or someone else?

- Percentage of the heart condition caused by self versus interference, such as curses, bindings, cords, hauntings, or assumption of others' energies, beliefs, and feelings.

- Vibration of your harmonic. Heart conditions involve tissues that are out of tune with your core harmonic. What is your core harmonic?

- Vibration of the chakra. What is the correct vibration of your primary disease chakra site? If this site is different than the heart, also examine for the correct heart chakra vibration.

- Vibration of the master diseased cells. What frequencies are they holding? How is that affecting the surrounding cells and organs?

- What holds the heart condition in place? What data is instructing your body to hold on to this disease? Is there an issue within the corresponding chakra?

- Sources. Are there sources, such as energies or beings, either inside or outside of you, keeping the heart problem locked in place?

- Information from your subconscious. What is the message your inner self is trying to give you? Is it about love?

- Information from your spirit. What need might you really be trying to meet, as perceived by your spirit and the Divine's spirit?

7. Create a statement of need that summarizes your conclusions in a few sentences.

Part Two: Healing Steps

After creating an energy map and an understanding of what initiated the heart problem, review your work, paying special attention to your statement of need. You will now prepare a plan of action, considering the following issues—again, this will be done more specifically on each pathway.

- Overall need
- Help that you can draw upon, both visible and invisible
- Spins that will meet the need
- Colors that will meet the need
- Tones that will meet the need
- Symbols that will meet the need
- Interference and connections to release
- Connections to make externally
- Connections to make internally
- Connections to make to other aspects of the self
- Reasons to release the heart problem
- Ways to meet the need differently through behavior, emotional expression, attitude and thinking, spiritual understandings, relationship connections, or psychic activity
- Ways to release the "self" at the age at which the heart condition was developed or the reasons it began
- Ways to release energies (beings, energies, consciousness, cords, and the like) causing or enforcing the heart problem; ways to forgive others and the self for this occurrence
- Ways to heal the heart condition at its source. Will this involve moving to a different pathway?
- Ways to change the vibration of the heart issue, chakra, body, or aspect of self. Will this involve shifting to a new pathway to make the job easier?

- Ways to alter permanently the master disease cells. Will this take a shift to a different pathway?
- Ways to assume the beliefs that will bring forth the whole self. Will this take a pathway shift?
- Ways to allow your subconscious to allow healing. Will this take a pathway jump?
- Ways to allow your spirit to assert its healing authority. Will this necessitate a pathway shift?

At this point, you should have a better understanding of the possible reasons you have cardiovascular disease and the ways in which you could approach your healing with love, grace, and power.

Deciding among Pathways

The truth is, you can work with any pathway for change. As seen in the final questions under the healing steps of energy mapping, you can always leap off your current pathway to employ another.

In general, however, I have found people gravitate toward one pathway over another. This is a snapshot of what might work best for you, based on your assessment of the Psychic Style Quiz (page 104).

Pathway	Gifted Chakras	Qualities
Elemental	First, second, third, tenth	People strongest in these chakras tend to benefit most from using their material-driven, physical strengths in the here-and-now world.
Power	Fifth, eighth, eleventh	People most gifted in these chakras can best access the supernatural forces of this pathway.

Imagination	Fourth, sixth eighth, tenth	People with skills from these psychic centers usually excel on this pathway.
Divine	Third, seventh, ninth	Individuals with these spiritual inclinations can make good use of this pathway's divine inspirations.

Linking the Pathways: A Means of Moving Energies between Pathways

You link pathways through assuming your wholeness. Here is an exercise that will help you consciously control this process.

The real link between you and all the pathways is through your spiritual essence or whole self. Automatically, energy and change are transferred through all the pathways.

1. Select a chakra as a focus. This can be the chakra you've been working on for healing or any favorite chakra. Now determine which pathway you're currently standing on, or select one as a starting point.

2. The center of this chakra serves as an elevator shaft to all other chakras on all other pathways. You can do one of two things through this elevator:

   · Deliver information or energies to other pathways
   · Obtain information or energies from other pathways

3. Decide what you want to accomplish, then proceed.

4. Allow full integration on all pathways and inside yourself.

PART Two

chapter six

Shift Healing on the Elemental Pathway

A whole water pot will fill up from drinking drops of water. A wise man fills himself with good, just a little at a time.

—The Dhammapada, verse 122†

Travel the elemental pathway under these conditions:

- You strongly believe in conventional treatments but are open to some holistic methods.
- You know you need to change your beliefs or attitudes to really heal.
- You are willing to take action to heal from heart disease.
- You are a here-and-now, action-oriented person.
- You want to use the elemental pathway as a basis, then supplement your care with one of the other pathways.
- You most often rely on your first, second, third, or tenth chakras.

The Elemental Pathway: Drops in the Bucket of Life

If you have a problem, on this pathway you follow the path of reductionism to discover which droplet is contaminating the

†Buddha, Guatama, *The Dhammapada*, John Richards trans., http://eawc.evansville.edu/anthology/dhammapada.htm, accessed August, 2006, verse 122.

greater whole. The goal of *reductionism* is to analyze to the most basic cause of your heart issue, then to strategize from there. Essentially you must unearth the pattern causing the problem and the program causing the pattern. I call negative programs or patterns *contaminants*, because they pollute your natural goodness. You can then ask yourself a number of healing-oriented questions. Can you purge yourself of the contaminant? Erase it and start over again? Can you compensate or transmute the contaminant? Perhaps use a tool from another pathway? Look for the source of the problem and, as I suggested in chapter 3, you've found your solution.

There are two ideas that will make elemental healing faster, easier, and more effective. First, relinquish perfectionism for being "good enough." Believe in the strength of your intention and you will heal.

Second, dig for causes as deeply as you can. Here is a chart to help you find a place to start your search for the source of your heart problem. A *consciousness level* is a level or depth of awareness. A *heart level* references the type of heart-based issues regulated by a certain consciousness level, and a *brain level* refers to a brain system, which, in turn, operates a part of the body.

Levels of Heart Problems

Chakras	Consciousness Level	Heart Level	Brain Level	Main Issues	Key Points
1, 2, 8, 10, 11, 12	Subconscious	Low Heart (often the ventricles and electrical system)	Reptilian	Soul, inherited, conception	Primal, place of fear, shame, and core motivation: affect basis of health
1, 2, 3, 4, 5, 6, 12	Unconscious	Middle Heart (often the valves and basic circulatory system)	Mammalian	Mind, womb, early childhood	Thought-based, affects behavior

Chakras	Consciousness Level	Heart Level	Brain Level	Main Issues	Key Points
7, 8. 9, 11, 12	Consciousness	High Heart (often the atrial and magnetic systems)	Higher brain	Spiritual, inherited or learned	Sets perceptions about higher truths, such as love and joy

There are several chakras that interface with more than one consciousness level, but for the most part, the lower the chakra in relation to the body, the deeper the consciousness level. Your *subconscious* is your deepest and most basic level of awareness, usually programmed by your soul during preconception with your own fear and shame-based issues, as well as those acquired from your family system. You activate or interject negative issues because you think they will keep you safe. These negative issues in turn program your *Low Heart*, which is geographically associated with the ventricles and electrical system. The Low Heart stimulates your flight and fear reactions. Most acute and chronic heart conditions originate here, in the most primal aspect of the self. Organs housed within the most affected chakras refuse positive entrainment with the heart; they are out of syncopation with the rest of your body. The heart might not originate your subconscious issues, but it can be the victim of them, which is why it's important to locate the core disease chakra.

Working at this subterranean level is difficult, for your subconscious will resist healing. However, if you assert divine love and forgiveness into the subconscious, you can heal just about anything. Fear and shame might originate your basic health programs, but locked into the subconscious is also the ability to recognize and receive love.

Your *unconscious* is usually a reflection of your mind. Your unconscious connects to your *Middle Heart*, which physically operates the valves and some parts of the circulatory system. The Middle Heart is most affected by your mammalian brain or limbic system, which governs emotions, reasoning, and actions.

Most heart-healing programs aim at this level, informing you of what to eat, what supplements to take, and to quit smoking. The problem is that words can't get to the unconscious strongholds that create negative behaviors, and certainly they can't reach the subconscious programs underneath!

Your *consciousness* is tied to your spirit. The conscious self is able to tap into your *High Heart*, which is encoded with the spiritual values or genetics of your spirit, including concepts such as faith, truth, justice, hope, and love. The High Heart is associated with the atrial chambers and magnetics of the heart, and is fundamentally able to magnetize energies to you. It relates to the higher brain, which controls your perceptions and spiritual nature. Incorrect spiritual perceptions, often learned in childhood, carried from past lives, or acquired from religion or culture, can block the natural flow of ideas from our spirit to our heart and brain, usually resulting in positive or neutral conditions in certain chakras. The result can be a split between the highest aspect of your consciousness and your subconscious. Atrial fibrillations are often an attempt of the spirit to reach deeper into the heart. Valvular problems can indicate resistance of the mind. Ventricular problems can reveal resistance of the subconscious to divine love. The long, slow buildup of plaque follows an attempt of the Middle Heart to compensate for lack of spirit and High Heart.

Working with the elemental pathway will be far easier if you can picture the relationship among these very basic aspects of the heart and the overall self, and dig as deeply as you can for diagnosis and healing. If you have to choose between two possible disease chakras with which to work, select the one that operates more deeply.

Heart Disease on the Elemental Pathway

You can work with either conventional or holistic viewpoints on the elemental pathway. On the pathways, you:

- Assume wholeness rather than brokenness.
- Select healing activities that bring wholeness to the surface, rather than just fix the brokenness.
- Invoke a two-way transfer of energy, such as between your whole self and elemental self, between the elemental self and the self on any other pathway, or between the Greater Self and the elemental self.

The following tools for healing on the elemental pathway help you accomplish all three goals.

Using Intention to Invite Wholeness

We employ intention to produce dynamic change on the elemental pathway. An *intention* is a quality or state of mind formed around a purpose. Make a decision to set your intention and you are halfway to your goal!

Using Energies That Reside on the Elemental Pathway

There are many energy bodies on the elemental pathway; they separate into *managing energy bodies* and *secondary energy bodies*. Each regulates a physical, emotional, mental, spiritual, relational, or psychic set of concerns. The complete list is available in my book *Advanced Chakra Healing*; here, I will present only a few. I will then discuss practical applications. Remember to work first with your primary disease chakra, then with your secondary disease chakra. If you are confused, begin with your heart chakra or work with the chakra most related to your subconscious.

The Chakras Changes made within a chakra are also transferred to all areas of concern regulated by that chakra, as well as to other chakras on this and other pathways.

The Spiritual Points There are twenty of these higher chakra points in your broader energy field. They connect your elemental pathway with your divine self and back again into your body through your vertebrae. You can learn more about them in my books *Advanced Chakra Healing*, as well as *New Chakra Healing*.

The Auric Field The auric field provides structure, screening, and protection. Paired with the chakras, each auric band is responsible for communicating that chakra's needs to the world and for attracting energies from the world to meet those needs. I advise working with the auric bands associated with your primary and secondary disease site.

The Morphogenetic Fields Morphogenetic fields are great for diagnosing issues, especially if you are working with any of the chakras affected by the subconscious. By psychically viewing them through the tenth auric band, you can perceive ancestral, soul-related, or societal issues. You can also examine for curses, bindings, cords, and other entity interference, as well as environmental and food-related causes of cardiovascular disease. Treat the problem within your primary chakra site and transfer changes to other chakras as well as to the corresponding auric band(s).

The Energy Egg The inner layer of the energy egg is most closely associated with the elemental pathway, and so I stress it in this section. Through the inner layer you can determine which chakra is primary and attune to the elemental cause of the heart problem.

To view this layer, center yourself either in your pituitary gland or pineal gland. Through the pituitary gland, you can best perceive the actual events, feelings, beliefs, or beings that initiated your heart problem. When skilled at psychic vision, you can actually watch a rerun of causal situations, then rewrite the past to heal the problem.

Through the pineal gland, you will see or sense white, gray, black, or red energies in your body or in any of the chakras. These colorations distinguish levels of consciousness (or spiritual advancement) as well as the mix of negative, positive, and neutral energies.

Negative energies show as black and indicate the need to perform regressive or emotion-based healing. Positive energies appear off-white and point to spiritual misperceptions, which may respond to futuring techniques. Red reflects neutrons holding fear or shame-based messages, which must be altered to love-based messages. Gray shows a mixture of negative and positive charges. The chakra that appears most affected or discontent is probably your primary disease site.

When performing healing, you can journey within the egg's inner layer while visualizing healing choices. If you desire, access spiritual forces through the power pathway or spiritual waves in the third layer of the energy egg to make changes. (Chapter 7 discusses ways to work with spiritual forces and chapter 9 describes divine pathway practices.) You can use the second layer of the energy egg to perceive imagination pathway choices and translate a solution into your body.

The Etheric Mirror The etheric mirror, or Christ body, supports your spiritual purpose and life plan. It contains a blueprint for your perfect body. To infuse your body with its correct template, establish beams of white light between your primary or secondary disease chakras and the same areas in the etheric mirror, which will look just like those regions in your body, except healthy. Initiate a spin from the etheric mirror to transfer energy from that body into the physical body.

The Akashic Records The Akashic Records are an energy "organ" that records everything you have ever done, said, thought, or felt, across time. It also can show you possible futures.

Although you can access the Akashic Records through any chakra, it is easiest through your eighth chakra, which is the seed of your soul and karmic knowledge. On the elemental pathway, center yourself in your eighth chakra and psychically connect with the Akashic Records. I like to picture them as a large book or a hallway of doors. Ask the Divine to turn to the page (or to take you through the door) that relates to your heart condition. As the scene unfolds, you can also correct the situation from there. If needed, request that divine guidance take you into the future to show you what will eventually heal your heart.

The Shadow Records Whereas the Akashic Records reflect your "reality," the Shadow Records store everything that you could have become.

Among chakras, the heart center is most susceptible to regret, the belief that you've lost your chance to love. Believing this illusion has cast many a heart into despair, trauma, and disease. If your heart disease is negatively charged, the belief may involve regret. To find out, journey through your eighth chakra and psychically concentrate on the primary chakra site. Don't focus on the chakra itself; rather, look at the energy around it. It will appear translucent. This is the Shadow Record. Ask this Record to come alive so you can perceive the situation or issue that is creating the heaviness—and disease—in the heart. When healing, make sure you use the Forgiveness Exercise found in the Special Insert or the exercise Reading the Book of Life for a Heart Healing in chapter 7.

You can also use the Shadow Records to make treatment decisions. Think of a potential treatment, then look into the shadow area around the primary chakra site for a response.

Healing the Physical Body: The Basis of Elemental Healing

The elemental pathway is essentially physical. Through the elemental pathway, you can connect with the subconscious, shift between tachyons and quarks, and transfer energies at will through the chakras. I offer elemental pathway approaches to support the two most common traditional treatments for heart disease.

Surgery

Here are a number of elemental pathway methods to boost your recovery from cardiovascular surgery.

1. Consult with a nutritionist in advance. Create a dietary and supplement-based program for pre- and post-surgery.

Consult with your physician about these supplement recommendations, as some supplements and herbs are counterproductive to surgery. Consider a heart-healthy diet whenever possible.

2. Emphasize pink and gold. Pink is the color of human love and gold, of divine grace. Days before your surgery, begin imagining both colors throughout your auric field. Just before surgery, visualize these same colors brightening the area surrounding the part of your body that will be incised, the surgical room, and the surgical team.

3. During or after surgery, play music (classical is good) that beats 60 to 90 beats a minute. Studies show that music that mirrors the heartbeat is both healing and calming.

4. Deal with your emotional issues. Surgery stirs up the strongholds that underlie a heart condition. You will repair faster physically if you "do your work" beforehand. Additionally, the surgery will probably dredge up further issues, memories, and feelings. Prepare for this by lining up a therapist or trusted advisor to help you.

5. At the quanta level, two objects never touch. At the subatomic level, you aren't being cut. Fill the space in and around your injury site, before and after the surgery, with pink and gold or with spiritual waves from the divine pathway.

You might also consider nonsurgical alternatives that have shown great promise in recent studies. In *Heal Your Heart with EECP*, Dr. Debra Braverman details how patients with heart disease have been successfully treated using enhanced external counterpulsation (EECP). This FDA- and Medicare-approved procedure is scientifically validated, safe, noninvasive, and painless. Treatment with EECP involves using blood pressure cuffs to move blood through the body, which leads to the creation of new blood vessels that restore healthy blood flow to the heart. Remember to consult with your physician before undergoing alternative procedures.

Medication

All medications produce harmful side effects, especially for the liver and kidney. A holistic practitioner such as a naturopath or nutritionist can select a nutritional or supplement protocol to compensate.

I frequently program medication for my clients. This involves tapping into the divine pathway and asking the Divine to align the medicine's ingredients for my client's well-being.

It's also helpful to work with the elements, which are referenced later in this chapter. Consider using metal to protect the kidney and liver from toxic damage; water to flush the body of poisons; wood to achieve pH homeostasis; and fire to burn away toxic residues.

As with all elemental pathway healing, intention will bring about the desired results.

Set the inner wheel of your primary disease chakra, your liver, and your kidneys in reverse so they can spin the toxins out of your body. You can also set the eighth chakra's inner wheel in reverse, as well as the eighth auric band, in order to cleanse your body.

Check, too, that you have a positive spin on your lymph system and nodes, so they can carry out toxins generated by the standard treatments. You can use generative or degenerative spiritual forces from the power pathway to amplify any of these procedures.

Basic Life Needs and the Chakras

Basic life needs are regulated by particular chakras, as follows:

- Shelter: Tenth (environment) and first (clothing)
- Breathing: Tenth (environment) and fourth (lungs)
- Water: First (skin), fifth (drinking), and all other in-body chakras
- Touch: First (skin and genital entry points) and fifth (eating)

- Movement: All
- Food: All

Work with these chakras in the following ways to assist with healing.

Shelter That Heals Your tenth chakra forges your relationship with nature and the environment. In order to create a healing environment to support your subconscious, use your psychic perception to center in your tenth chakra, then think of each of the following categories:

- Plants, trees, and flowers
- Fountains or bowls of water
- Stones, rocks, and crystals
- Colors, fabrics, and textures
- Music and sounds

What substances seem to support your well-being, turn your home into a healing haven, or lift your heart? Once you establish these items in your home, ask the Divine to open your tenth chakra to the beneficial healing properties the item carries, then imagine a white light connecting your heart or primary disease chakra to the object.

If your heart problems involve "attacks on your heart," either from animate or inanimate beings, use oil or sage smoke to mark the windowsills and doorways with the symbol of a cross within a circle, thus sealing your home against potentially harmful energies.

Different stones and rocks carry different properties that can bring helpful healing energy. You can put these stones in your home or wear them as jewelry. For heart protection, I recommend obsidian or amethyst. For heart healing, try fluorite or tourmaline. For love, use pink quartz or jade. For heart hormone balancing, wear ruby or garnet (especially helpful as earrings).

Metal, too, can make a difference. Silver offers protection against negative people and entities, and it also serves as a conduit for higher guides. Yellow gold carries the vibration of your etheric mirror and induces good health and a healthy perspective, while white gold upholds the spiritual in the practical. Copper cleanses the blood, and platinum increases spiritual awareness.

Remember that color, fabric, and metals are made of energy. Center yourself in your first chakra and think of various colors and clothing items. Choose colors, fabrics, and styles that ease your heart and support your intention.

The Power of Breath Your lungs and heart are physically very close together and are integral friends. I recommend connecting these two organs energetically with your tenth chakra, which works like a second set of lungs inside of the earth, thus supporting the elimination of toxins into the ground and the acceptance of earth energies into your body. A helpful exercise is to imagine that your subconscious self rests down in your tenth chakra and is ready to be healed in support of your heart health. Every time you breathe in, you are receiving the Divine's Spirit. Every time you breathe out, you are allowing the Spirit to eliminate toxins, diseases, and old issues. Now concentrate on your breath. During the in-breath, receive the Divine and ask it to link your lungs, heart, and tenth-chakra subconscious with love. During your exhalation, allow the Divine to release you from the issues causing you distress and illness. Do this exercise anytime.

Smoking is one of the key indicators of developing heart disease. I find that most people smoke for emotional reasons. A cigarette is a companion. Smoke covers up our inner loneliness. It serves as a smokescreen to our gifts. Think back to when you started smoking and why. What was going on in your life? You're still smoking for the same reasons. Deal with the emotions, and it will be much easier to quit. I also suggest acupuncture and nutritional supplementation as a vital part of the process.

And don't forget laughter—it releases endorphins and lightens the heart.

Cleansing through Water Your body is more than 75 percent water. Water can easily be programmed for healing by using the following method. Simply hold your hands over your glass of water or beverage, and ask the Divine to change the molecules into powerful healing particles. Superimpose a power pathway force into your beverage to support this request, or use the imagination pathway processes to imagine the life you desire while drinking. Consider also drinking out of a bottle upon which you've written your dreams and goals or healing words, such as "faith" and "love."

Awakening through Touch Touch affects the first auric band and chakra. Research shows a strong correlation between the skin and the heart; a healthy and loving touch eases the heart. Unless your doctor orders otherwise, continue a sensual or sexual life with a loving partner. Get a massage. Sleep with a baby blanket, a soft stuffed animal, or better yet, your animal companion.

Exercising to Endear Your Heart One of the leading causes of heart disease is lack of exercise; conversely, exercise is one of the most healing techniques. Different types of exercise alter the spin of your energy organs, physical organs, and individual cells. Consider selecting an exercise that promotes the greatest positive spin in your primary chakra site. Here are examples of various activities and the chakras they affect.

- *Walking:* Primarily heart and secondarily all other chakras. Excellent for building connection among all organs, as walking creates a flow of energy among the chakras. If you focus on a spiritual point when walking, you invite its force more deeply into your body.
- *Running:* First, heart, and tenth chakras. Set the goal of cleansing your subconscious while running.
- *Biking:* First, heart, and tenth chakras. Think "freedom" for your subconscious while peddling; that is, freedom from all issues causing your heart disease.

- *Swimming:* Primarily second and secondarily all other chakras. Water replicates the water of life, emotions, and psychic well-being. Swim to release pent-up feelings and others' feelings, and to integrate spiritual energies into your spine.
- *Tennis and racquetball:* Primarily first and secondarily all other chakras. Excellent for eleventh and twelfth chakras. If playing singles, concentrate on inviting your subconscious to release its power issues. If playing doubles, focus on releasing subconscious issues regarding relationships.
- *Downhill skiing:* All chakras. Ensures flow under adversity. Concentrate on bonding your wounded chakra/subconscious with nature and speed—speed for healing, that is.
- *Weightlifting:* Primarily eleventh and secondarily all other chakras. If your heart issues are related to power issues (as in negatively charged heart diseases, weightlifting can be very empowering).
- *Yoga:* First and seventh chakras. Excellent for integration of the entire body. Yoga encourages serpent and golden kundalini (discussed in chapter 7) to align your body-based subconscious and unconscious self with your conscious, higher self.
- *Martial arts:* Primarily first, second, sixth, seventh, eighth, and eleventh chakras, secondarily all remaining chakras. Increases life energy and connects spiritual energies with physical strengths. Establishes a discipline of higher chakras and the higher self over lower chakras and the lower self.
- *Dancing:* Primarily fourth and secondarily all other chakras. Expresses your spirit through your body.

Fueling Life through Food

Besides water, food is the most important healing substance you can use physically. When combined with chakra healing, food can take on medicinal value.

A few factors to consider include pH balance; metabolic disruptors and assistants; foods for primary chakra sites; and the role of the elements. After considering these four areas, we'll examine the complex arena of diet supplementation. My goal isn't to offer medical or professional advice; it is to show you how to work with informed vibration through the chakras to gain optimal benefit from whatever plan you adopt. More detailed information and techniques are available in my book *Advanced Chakra Healing.*

Foods and pH balance: The pH measurement, on a scale of 0 to 14, indicates the balance between acidity and alkalinity in your body. It can be measured using body fluids. Many holistic practitioners believe urine reflects physical issues and saliva shows the presence of emotional issues.

A reading lower than 7.0 reflects more acidity; a reading higher than 7.0 indicates more alkalinity. Many nutritionists and holistic practitioners suggest 7.4 as an ideal level, because it is easier for the body to oxygenate when in a slightly alkaline condition. When working with the elemental pathway, I recommend you work with a professional to test your pH balance frequently. Use your urine to monitor diet and supplements and your saliva to note mental and emotional strongholds. I usually find that alkaline conditions indicate positive-charged issues, while acidic measurements reveal negative-charged issues. A neutral issue can underlie either. Your body can be a combination of both.

In general, you can sustain a healthy pH balance by abstaining from all white foods, which include milk, yeast, white flours, and sugar. Also consider eliminating fruits with simple sugars, white potatoes and rice, corn, coffee, soda pop, alcohol, fruit juices, cheese, junk food, processed soy products, processed meats, high-salt foods, mushrooms, pork, store-bought sauces, hydrogenated or trans fats, saturated fats, foods with aspartame, foods with hormones, foods with chemical preservatives, and animal meats high in fat, such as red meat. For the most part, caffeine should be excluded, as should MSG and other stimulants. Restrict alcohol to no more than two ounces of red wine a day, although you can get the same benefit from red grape juice. Also consider restricting your use of "healthy" foods high in saturated fats, such as avocados, nuts, seeds, and most animal products. Use salt moderately. Allowed are teas, which are very heart-healthy, egg whites, and yogurt. Consider sculpting an eating program using the concepts in my book, *Attracting Your Perfect Body through the Chakras*, which enables a personalized approach to health and fitness.

It's very difficult to eat perfectly, and I don't think you have to. Indulge in your favorite foods once in a while. In the Four Pathways approach, there's more to food than the substance of it.

Whatever encodes to a particular food encodes to you and can create cravings, dislikes, and physiological effects. At the end of the food section, I provide an easy-to-use exercise for breaking the bonds between nutrients and harmful energies.

Metabolic disruptors and assistants: A *metabolic disruptor* is any substance or nutrient that stops or derails the normal function of your cells and organs. A *metabolic assistant* creates or supports the healthy functioning of your cells and organs. All metabolic food agents fit into one of these four categories: fats, sugars, proteins, and liquids. Other categories include vitamins, minerals, enzymes, and other elements. In pathway healing, the energy charging a substance is just as important as the actual substance, if not more so. Any substance can be charged with energy; the following is a guide.

- Negative spins make the substance decrease power or energy. These substances will make you tired, trigger old strongholds, and empower a sad subconscious. Body areas affected by these substances will tend toward an acidic condition, including an attraction to viruses. To compensate, the body might eventually attract "positive" energies to reverse the spin, such as bacteria or yeast, possibly leading to Candida, which disrupts the heart entrainment with first-, second-, or third-chakra organs.

- Positive spins cause substances to reject love or spiritual energies. These nutrients spin out of the body, and you'll experience deficits in regard to these nutrients or properties.

- An absence of spins where there should be spins can make a strong misperception attach to a nutrient and cancel out its healthy properties. Over time, enough "neutered" energies can make your chakras stop moving.

- Interference, such as an entity, consciousness, or energetic contract, can disrupt healthy frequencies and can lead to bad habits and cravings, as the organ seeks balance.

Refer to the exercises at the end of this food section to break harmful nutritional bonds and support your nutrients energetically.

Primary chakra sites and related foods: In general, you can boost the healing power of your healthy tissue governed by the primary disease chakra by feeding the healthy tissue foods that vibrate at the same rate. It's important first to charge these foods with helpful information, so that they become healing foods. To choose the right foods for you, see my books *Advanced Chakra Healing* and *Attracting Your Perfect Body through the Chakras.*

Supplements: It is best to consult a professional for a customized assessment of supplements. Depending upon your primary disease chakra, I suggest you research for your particular chakra type. Also consider the use of homeopathic medicine, Bach Flower Remedies, and other vibrational medicines, if specifically customized to your condition.

Following is a list of heart-healthy supplements to consider. Doctors almost universally recommend a good multivitamin that contains B_{12}, iron, and trace minerals. You can also work with a naturopath or nutritionist to diagnose deficiencies in vitamin C, vitamin B, vitamin B3, vitamin B6, vitamin B12, folate, magnesium, vitamin D (if not getting enough sun), selenium, CoQ10, or vitamin E. Be careful with vitamin B3, also called niacin; in certain people, it can have negative side effects, as can vitamin E. Consider using heart supplements that include alpha lipoic acid, red yeast rice, garlic, soy protein, extra fiber, hawthorn, cumin, turmeric, garlic, green tea, white tea, black tea, and omega oils. There are two opposing thoughts about supplementing with fish oil. Many fish oils contain mercury and are rancid. Because of this, many professionals recommend using other forms of omega-3s, such as those that are vegetarian-based.

Exercises to Energize Food for Healing

Here are two exercises to connect informed vibration to food for healing.

The "Unbonding" Exercise This exercise will free nutrients and inorganic and organic compounds from harmful programs, interference, and bad charges. You can use this for all food properties, liquids, additives, elements, and metabolic disruptors.

1. Center in the sense, feeling, or awareness that results from ingesting a problem food. You may or may not know exactly which element or compound is causing the problem. Acknowledge that something is disturbing your digestive health.

2. Ask to see, hear, or sense which chakra is most affected by this element or compound, then bring your attention to this chakra.

3. Ask to perceive the element or compound causing difficulties. Now immediately ask to perceive the energy that is bonded to this property and triggering bodily reactions.

4. Request information about this harmful bond. What do you need to understand? What caused its inception? How is this bond affecting you? Is it primarily related to a belief, a feeling, a spin, or an interference? Now ask what you need to do

or to understand to fully and permanently release this harmful bond.

5. Release the bond.

6. Ask which energies you need to activate from deep inside or receive from outside to fill in the gap, to cleanse the bodily area of built-up negative effects, to create a positive relationship with this energy, and to strengthen or reinforce the helpful energies of this or any other physical element or compound.

7. Check for spin. Are there any changes you now need to transfer into the primary chakra site? Coordinate spin and energies between the property and the chakra, and then close.

Exercise for Fortification You can select any food, supplement, herb, homeopathic remedy, liquid, or product and boost its helpful qualities. You can do the same for medicines. Here is an exercise for fortifying a substance in your body. This is a way to create a metabolic assistant.

1. Hold the thought, tone, sense, or picture of the selected property in your mind. Ask which chakra vibrates closest to this property's frequency. Bring your consciousness into that chakra.

2. Ask to perceive the energy that will increase the positive and helpful effects of this property in your body in light of your chosen goal. State your goal. Now visualize, sense, or hear a symbol, a color, a light, an element, a number, a tone, a spin, or any other marker that you will now attach to this property.

3. At what intensity, speed, and spin should this property vibrate to accomplish your goal? If it is supporting a toxic element or compound, ask for an "energy container" so that the element will accomplish only the established goal.

4. Ask the Divine to bless this process and alert you when it's done.

The Role of the Elements

The entire physical universe breaks down to ten major elements: water, earth, air, fire, metal, wood, stone, ether, light, and star. Imbalances of any of these elements can create the vibrational disturbances that cause or support heart disease; conversely, using or balancing these elements can correct heart conditions.

Working with the elements can be done physically or psychically. When working with elements physically, consider consulting with a professional such as an oriental medicine expert, an energy worker, or a naturopath to assess for missing, imbalanced, or congested elements. These can then be matched to the appropriate chakric healing techniques, supplements, or dietary changes to address the situation. When working with elements psychically, assess for problems with elements and make the necessary corrections using your primary intuitive style. You can also employ a professional energy healer or ask a spiritual guide for help.

Here are the basic properties of the ten elements:

- *Fire:* Eliminates, purges, and burns away. Use fire to purify the blood, lymph system, clotted areas, and plaque. Do not use directly on the heart, as fire can enhance anger and inflammation.
- *Air:* Transmits ideas and ideals. Use it to "blow away" bad beliefs or initiate helpful ones.
- *Water:* Transmits psychic and feeling energies, soothes and heals, washes and cleanses. Use to cleanse your lymph system or intestines of toxins, both psychic and physical; to purify the body from old and repressed feelings (of the self or others); and to calm tissues after surgery. Wash a stroke site with water, then build an earth or a stone wall around the site while healing. Also consider programming your drinking water, as explained in the Cleansing through Water section (see page 183).

- *Earth:* Builds, solidifies, and protects. Earth can rebuild tissue after surgery, soothe any inflamed area, and repair tissues, such as valves. Use it after washing a stroke site with water to help reconstruct tissue.
- *Metal:* Protects, defends, and deflects. Use it in the auric field to deflect harmful energies. Establish a metal energetic fort around the liver or kidneys if you are taking medication (this will also draw heavy-metal toxicity out of these organs). Use it as a temporary armor around your heart or any other organ being attacked from external energies or entities.
- *Wood:* Adds buoyancy, adaptability, and a positive attitude. Insert it in areas of depressed or counterclockwise spin to help set the spin to clockwise. If you are depressed emotionally, add it to the mind. Use wood to integrate new tissue or ideas into the body, such as after surgery to assist in the body's acceptance of a stent or pacemaker. If you have high blood pressure, consider adding wood psychically or keeping wood within close physical proximity for relaxation. Oriental medicine practitioners frequently work with wood and might be especially beneficial.
- *Stone:* Strengthens, holds, and toughens. Use stone in the tenth chakra to keep the soul grounded in the body. Replace soul/subconscious shame with stone to provide strength. Add stone to a weak blood vessel or around a stroke site by using supplements recommended by a professional or by psychically imagining stone. It helps to think of stone as a safe fortress, which will then calm anxiety. Stone will hold other elements in place; if you need to keep new beliefs anchored so they can root, build a stone retaining wall to do so.
- *Ether:* Holds spiritual truths; can be used to infuse any system, energy body, mind, or soul with such spiritual truths. Use it to bring spiritual truths from the divine pathway into the physical body. Ether will integrate spirit, High Heart, and the higher brain truths into the heart or any other organ.

Use during atrial or ventricular palpitations to bring healing truths. To use ether elementally, concentrate on the primary symptom or chakra site and ask yourself or the Divine to psychically indicate the spiritual truth or awareness that can heal the underlying issue, then invoke the healing powers of love. Psychically infuse the problematic area with this insight and ask that the Divine distribute it to all levels of your being.

· *Light:* Can be directed, spun, fashioned, summoned, or eliminated to produce almost any desired effect. It is especially helpful for electrical or magnetic imbalances. Light is electromagnetic radiation of various wavelengths. Dark light is composed mainly of electrons that carry intelligence about power; "light" light is fashioned chiefly from protons that hold intelligence about love. Bring balance to any off-spin with the correct light. Use white, gold, or pink light to bring divine love into the subconscious, the soul, the ventricles, or the heart as a whole.

· *Star:* Uses spiritual truths to form and purify physical matter. Use star to burn a spiritual truth into your tissue to reprogram strongholds, change a power field, or alter DNA. Star will also force the release of a misperception or harmful pattern in the body. Use star when burning away an inaccurate perception in any consciousness level, then stimulate correct beliefs with ether. (Star is made of fire and ether; by intuitively mixing ether and fire, you create star.) To perform healing with star, concentrate on the primary symptom or chakra site and consider the belief that is causing the issue. Ask yourself what new or positive idea would correct the problem. Imagine what this chakra would look, feel, sound, or seem like if this idea were to take root and promote healing. Decide that this idea will not only heal your chakra and the corresponding illness but your entire being. Now clear away all images, sounds, and other sensory perceptions; what remains is the ether, or ethereal basis, of your healing. Ask the Divine to burn this ether, which carries the solution to your health, into your primary chakra point with the fire of star. Share this star energy with all other chakras and distribute throughout your body to complete the healing.

Working with Strongholds

The basis of most elemental pathway healing involves breaking strongholds. You might really want to change a pattern but find yourself unable to do so because the energy of the stronghold binds you in place. Here are initial ways to free your feelings and beliefs. If these don't work, move to the next sections of this chapter and assess the situation for interference, and time and space issues. You can also work directly with energy techniques or consider moving to the power pathway, where more intense energies might be holding you.

Freeing Your Feelings Most negatively based heart problems involve repressed feelings. You can energetically determine the presence and placement of harmful feelings by looking for counterclockwise spins; squared-off symbols; dark or bluish energies; and heavy-feeling areas in the body, energy organs, or auric bands.

Also, the second chakra records feelings for the entire system. Examine the back of the second chakra, looking for discolorations, off-marks, off-tones, or other indications of stored energies. Dark energy lines, which are actually internal cords, will track to the entry or storage site of these feelings. Assess the inner wheel of the second chakra. If it is clearly spinning in reverse, either this or another chakra is holding repressed feelings. These feelings may have originated with you, others, or both.

Before you can work with your own feelings, eliminate others' energies using the releasing exercises Freeing Yourself from Others' Energies and Interference in the Special Insert. Center yourself in your primary disease chakra, then use the Healing Feelings exercise in the Special Insert to release the feeling, determine its message, and undo the stronghold.

Healing Your Beliefs Destructive beliefs come from the past. You may have personally determined them or simply absorbed them from others. Harmful beliefs are primarily stored in the electrons—which initiate structure—and therefore these beliefs affect your sense of power. In cases involving negative heart conditions, which will most likely lie in the subconscious and perhaps unconscious, your life is designed around these harmful beliefs. In cases of positive heart problems, which are more apt to affect the unconscious and the conscious, the programming in the protons determines your ability to give and receive love. If your beliefs discount the importance of love, your own body won't love itself enough to heal your heart or allow it health. Neutron-based heart problems involve a single belief, which establishes a universal pattern that affects all of your life. Change the belief creating the heart problem, and you can change your entire life.

Hurtful beliefs can eventually erode healthy physical and energetic systems. Inserting healthy and loving beliefs into our chakras, bodies, minds, and cells can enable positive restructuring and genetic reprogramming.

Here is a simple exercise to alter a belief-based pattern. Conduct it after you have determined whether or not you are currently taking on beliefs from others, as discussed in the insert.

Exercise for Changing Your Beliefs

1. Center yourself in the chakra holding the originating belief or belief stronghold. You can always track energy lines through the back of the fourth chakra to the conflicted chakra, if it differs from the fourth. Now view through the seventh chakra's pineal gland, where you will observe dark, light, or red energies in all chakras that show strongholds.

Dark indicates an electron (negative) basis; off-white, a proton (positive) basis; and red, a neutron basis. Gray is a mixture of negative and positive. Additionally, check for spin and color in various chakras. Dark and reverse spins reveal electrons and probably emotional strongholds; light and clockwise spins indicate protons and, typically, mental strongholds; red and stuck spins mean neutrons and a single, foundational misperception.

2. Use the table of power levels and fields in my book *Advanced Chakra Healing* to get a sense of which types of beliefs are causing problems. Refer to the listing of beliefs in the Special Insert (under Energy Absorption Issues) to help define your harmful beliefs.

3. Ask your intuition or the Divine to clarify the original misperception or set of beliefs causing the stronghold. You will hear, sense, or see an answer. Ask to understand the origin of the belief. At what age did you initiate or accept this belief? In which lifetime? For what reason? What contract is keeping this belief in place? Are you holding this agreement with another person or energy, or primarily with yourself?

4. Ask now what you need to understand or do to release the misperceptions and initiate a helpful belief. The beliefs you are meant to have are based on spiritual truths.

Basic Energy Healing: Special Techniques for the Elemental Pathway

Elemental pathway healing involves basic concepts of working energetically. By reducing your diagnosis to electrical or negative, positive or magnetic, neutron or neutral, you can tap into the world of informed vibration and use the following concepts for healing: particles and waves, spin, color, form, tones, forces, and fields. Included in this section are exercises for improving the success of traditional treatments.

Particle and Wave Healing Recall that particles can turn into waves, and vice versa. Waves generate a much stronger field than do particles. The heart operates through oscillating waveforms, forming cross-coherent patterns with other organs that do the same. Use these facts to your advantage in the following ways.

- Toxic or damaged cells are particles, though they can emanate waves throughout your body. With intention, chakra-based meditation, use of vibrational medicines such as homeopathy, or programmed music, you can disempower toxins, harmful hormones, negative side effects of medication, bad fats, or other harmful substances by calling forth a wave from your own spirit. This second wave will harmonize to your body and will naturally be more powerful than any subversive energy.

- Healthy cells are particles. Their energetics, however, can be transformed into a waveform. Use intention to free a healthy cell's energy, so it works like a wave. Intensify this wave and direct it at discordant heart energies.

- Many negative heart conditions are linked to viruses, which, in turn, link to group consciousness waves. To deal directly with an underlying virus, call forth a spiritual truth available on the divine pathway or through a spiritual point. Turn this truth into a wave to eliminate the virus.

- Many positive heart problems are connected with yeast, mold, and bacteria. When these grow in the body, they encourage the development of acidity, which then generates negative energies in the body. Yeast, mold, and bacteria exist in the presence of spiritual assumptions that are self-defeating and damaging. Psychically examine these microbes for the consciousness wave that carries the destructive ideas. Bring in a wave of truth to change the ideas.

- For potent healing of neutral heart issues, erase the harmful belief in the center of the cell or chakra that carries it. Substitute a wave of truth.

Spin Check the primary disease site for incorrect spin, then use your intuition to determine the correct spin. Once you've established the correct spin, lock it in with a symbol. You can select an appropriate symbol, number, or tone after conducting the chapter 7 exercise for discovering your harmonic. You also can always turn to the Divine to select a lock for you, or you can test a symbol psychically and see whether it holds.

Once you have altered your primary chakra, check all your other chakras and set their spins correctly. Check for the rhythm inside each chakra and between all chakras.

You can also alter the spins of diseased cells. Sometimes you have only to bring order to their erratic spins, and the heart's innate accuracy will take over and assist the healing.

One interesting technique for changing spins is to do so on X-rays, ECGs, MRIs, or scans instead of on the body. Hold your pendulum over the X-ray or scan to assess for spin. Use intention to change the pattern on your scan, then ask the Divine to transfer the necessary healing energies into your body to create this change permanently.

Color As described in the Special Insert, you can work with color diagnostically or for healing. Psychically, a healthy electron state is a deep rich ebony or a pretty blue. A negatively based heart problem will appear as an ugly black or muddy blue. You can always ask the Divine to provide you the correct hue of black when working with negative issues. Positive heart conditions usually appear a strange, milky white or off-yellow. Gold is the sign of healthy protons and a good color to work with for positive issues. Neutral heart problems will reflect red tones, but shades of pink or rose are the best to work with for healing these neutral heart problems.

Form Use the lists of forms in the Special Insert (under Evaluating Form) to evaluate the shapes in your primary chakra sites. If you've removed an unhealthy shape during your work, be sure to replace it with a new form. In general, circular shapes establish healthy relationships, square shapes offer protection, pyramid shapes restore the ability to manifest, and spirals create release or attraction. A cross with a circle is always a good shape for locking in a beneficial change.

Numbers can also be useful. Someone who is lonely will have a numeral 1 in his or her chakra centers. By simply substituting the numeral 2, you enable the person to attract partnership. With heart disease, you most frequently want to work with circular shapes and even numbers, both of which enhance relationships.

Tones If you are an auditory psychic, toning can be of great benefit. Determine your personal spiritual harmonic, as detailed in chapter 7. Once you know your harmonic, you'll intuitively know which tones are healthy for you and which ones are not.

In general, lower-frequency tones can help break up negative issues, higher-frequency tones can alter positive heart conditions, and middle-range tones can help reprogram neutral states. For potent toning, vibrate tones in octaves. This creates a harmonic that disrupts a distorted pattern on both sides.

Forces and Fields There are many types of natural forces. A complete list is outlined in my book *Advanced Chakra Healing*. Analyze which is fueling your heart problem. You can obtain the answer by working psychically in your primary disease chakra site. Now ask your spiritual guides or the Divine to tell you how to combat the relationship between the heart problem and the force. Select a force that will disrupt the harmful bond and insert another one that creates connection. You can always complement helpful natural forces with spiritual energetic forces from the power pathway (see chapter 7).

Here are a few ways to use personal fields, auric bands, external fields, and power fields for your healing process.

Personal Fields The heart emanates its own fields, and these mirror your harmonic or personal fields. Working with the electrical field can help you balance most negative heart conditions, and the same is true with the magnetic field and positive heart conditions. You can work with the entire electromagnetic field for most neutral conditions.

To assist in balancing your electrical field, first use techniques like regression or dealing with your feelings and old beliefs to uncover the underlying issue. You might need to perform physical procedures such as detoxification, diet changes, blessing of your water, or intense exercise. Be sure to consult with your primary heart physician to verify that these are safe for you. Then center yourself in your heart or primary disease chakra site, and ask the Divine to connect with your electrical field and to charge it correctly for your well-being. The same exercise will work for balancing your magnetic or overall electromagnetic field, after first performing healings pertinent to the charges in these fields.

Auric Bands In general, you work with the auric bands as you would with the chakras (see the insert for a full description of the auric field). Check for energetic contracts, possession or recession, absorption of other energies, and all other matters. Use regression, projecting, or futuring to define further the origination issues and vibrational means to heal. You may choose to attend to the following particular issues.

Holes: Auric holes allow in energies that are psychically or physically disruptive to your natural rhythms. Auric field holes related to your primary disease site are stealing your basic life energy and opening you to external toxins. When closing holes, make sure you first release any stored negative energies from the body.

Weak spots: Weakened, thin, light-colored, or soft auric areas illuminate weakened conditions in the corresponding chakras and related organs. Strengthen these weak spots with tonal or color therapy and lock the changes in symbolically.

Discoloration: You might spot colors that don't fit in this band, are muddied, or are otherwise disturbed. These off-hues mirror the conditions causing problems in the chakras. Some discolorations reflect the genetic abnormalities; if this is the case, access the spiritual genetics on the power pathway, as described in chapter 7. Then transfer these spiritual energies into your physical genes before fully correcting your auric field. Other discolorations are due to interjected energies from others. In this case, jettison others' energies before filling in with the correct color, tone, or symbol.

Symbology issues: Like the chakras, the auric bands can contain symbols. Look carefully to observe whether any of these representations are linked or corded to your primary disease site or injured body part. Change the symbol and establish a new one in the pertinent chakra and auric band.

Off-tones: The aurally gifted can hear the tones of the various auric bands and perceive variations. Listening to music in your own harmonic, chanting, or humming can change a discordant tone. You can even picture the correct note and insert it into the field. In the case of heart disease, an exceptionally gifted verbal psychic can ask to hear the symphony of the heart in relation to the rest of the body, and ask the Divine to establish this healing music throughout the entire auric field.

Interference: With few exceptions, interference that is obvious within a chakra will be visible within an auric band. You can work in either place to challenge and change this interference.

External Fields *Ley lines* are fields of electromagnetic energies in the earth. They are part of the family of *Vivaxis energies*—energetic lines and networks that connect all living things with electromagnetic energies found in and above the earth. Your family lineage might be corded to a ley line on unhealthy soil or on ancestral land that retains a charge that established a genetic formula for heart problems. If your heart issue is negative, consider that you may be hooked into a highly electrical ley line or another electrical field, such as those from a planet or a star. For positive heart problems, evaluate your energy fields for highly magnetic ley lines or other Vivaxis connections. Regarding neutral heart conditions, look to see whether you need to be connected to a certain type of electromagnetic line to activate your healing abilities.

Working in the Power Fields *Power fields* are a progressive order of energetic fields that stair-step you through the human development process into owning your divinity. A complete outline of power levels and power fields is available in *Advanced Chakra Healing*. Working with your power field is an exceptionally effective way to support your electromagnetic system and eliminate strongholds. To heal a stronghold energetically through power field work, see the information and exercises in *Advanced Chakra Healing*.

The Inner Child Asking for Rescue I am a strong believer in working through inner-child issues. Your inner children are aspects of the self that are still stuck in an earlier time because of trauma. Energetically, they continue to experience the initial tragedy until they are freed and healed.

The body will interpret an inner child and its feelings, beliefs, and corded energies as a foreign object, and it will either attack this inner child and create inflammation or build a wall of shame around it. This is one of the major causes of heart disease.

To perform inner-child work, you must first gain the trust of the hidden self and uncover his or her tale. You must then rescue this child, which will free your stuck energy and enable you to heal the part of the body that was secreting the child. An inner child is frequently involved in an emotional stronghold and sometimes in a mental stronghold. Inner-child work can be quite productive in physical healing because it is deep work. Inner children mirror soul issues, which lock into the subconscious, become fodder for unconscious beliefs, and

When you heal an inner child, you heal the soul and pave the way for attracting powerful spiritual energies that magnify healing.

create the schism between the spirit and your brain's consciousness. Although past-life trauma is sometimes the reason that a this-life child draws an experience into itself, no one is responsible for abuse suffered in a past life! Abusers are always responsible for their own actions. A soul trauma affects the energy system, leaving holes and strongholds that prevent you from knowing how to create safety.

Inner-Child Healing Here are the basic steps involved in reaching and helping an inner child:

1. Begin work in the primary disease chakra site. Check for indications of an inner child, as noted above.

2. Ask to communicate with this child. Have the child show you what occurred to cause the fear, emptiness, or shame. After receiving the story, ask the inner child how its presence has been affecting your life.

3. To help the child self, ask the child what is needed. Usually, the need is to be rescued from the threat, which, from the child's perspective, is still occurring. Call upon the Divine, guardian angels, or your own future or higher self to help address the threat.

4. Upon removing the child from the scene of the trauma, ask the Divine where this child needs to be kept so the child will be safe until "grown up." Cleanse the trauma site energetically or have a spiritual guide do it.

5. Check for cords, especially ones connected to the abuser. Also evaluate for codependent cords or life-energy cords to a past life. Use the cord exercise in the Special Insert to deal with these.

6. Establish the correct spin patterns in the chakra before closing.

For further assistance in inner-child healing, I recommend *The Inner Child Workbook* by Cathryn Taylor.

Dealing with Interference As explained in the Special Insert, *interference* is any form of energy or entity that keeps you from living in your own truth. Energetically, an interference establishes a vibration or set of vibrations that inhibit your own harmonic. When working on the elemental pathway, check the following places or sites for energetic contracts, entities, group consciousness, hauntings, or other types of interference, including areas in which you have absorbed others' energies.

- Chakras, auric bands, and other energy bodies
- Organs or regions affected by the heart disease
- The lymph system near primary or secondary disease sites
- Foods, supplements, or liquids commonly consumed
- Morphogenetic fields
- The inside layer of the energy egg or between the layers of the energy egg—interference between the first and second layer can prevent realization of your dreams for healing—and interference between the second and third layer can deflect healing spiritual energies
  - Any part or aspect of the self

If interference is present, use the exercises in the Special Insert section titled Freeing Yourself from Others' Energies and Interference to clear it.

Kundalini: The Serpent Rising In cases of heart disease, kundalini on the elemental pathway is nearly always erratic. Kundalini expresses itself as a serpent that rises through the body. It appears red, because it is composed of basic life energy. Frequently, red kundalini energy gets stuck in the first chakra, creating adrenal dysfunction, emotional repression, low self-esteem, and insufficient heart energy. Sometimes the red kundalini gets rewired directly from a lower chakra into the heart because of fears or blocks between the first and third chakras. In this case, it will inflame the heart and coronary arteries. Sometimes the kundalini jumps all the way to the head, where it pulses so strongly that it weakens blood vessels, thus leading to a stroke. In cases of thrombosis, embolisms, or aneurysms, sometimes the kundalini gets trapped in these regions, thus forming a real-life clot or bulge. You want your serpent kundalini to form a straight and even flow, from the first chakra in men and the second chakra in women, all the way up and around the body. Follow the exercises in my book *Advanced Chakra Healing* for working with your kundalini.

Time, Space, and Interdimensional Travels Sometimes heart disease is related to occurrences on other dimensions, time periods, or realms. With heart disease, I frequently find that aspects of the self are caught in the first or second dimensions for subconscious problems; third or fourth for unconscious issues; and fifth and above dimensions for conscious-based confusions. There are thirteen main dimensions, and it is best to access them through the eighth chakra or the heart, in the case of heart disease. You can also get to a dimension through the corresponding chakra. For instance, you can get to the fourth dimension through the fourth chakra.

To connect to another spacetime, use processes described in the Special Insert, such as the Projection Exercise or the Regression Exercise. Make sure you follow the insert's Five Steps for Safe Psychic Use. It's often easiest to conduct these types of connections through the eighth chakra or by using an imagination mirror on the imagination pathway (see chapter 8).

Here are various types of places and spaces. A complete description of these is available in my book *Advanced Chakra Healing*.

Planes of Light When the body dies, the soul passes through twelve planes to merge back into spirit. You can access the healing energies of any of these planes and transfer them into your current body at will. Read about the planes in *Advanced Chakra Healing*, then use Five Steps for Safe Psychic Use to conduct your travels.

Zones of Life and Death There are four zones that assist the soul in its alchemical processes between life, death, and the space in between lives. These can be especially helpful in working with the subconscious. You can access these zones through the eighth chakra or the primary disease chakra, or simply ask the Divine to connect you with any one of these zones. You can also use journeying techniques, such as regression, to recall your progression through any of these zones.

- *The White Zone:* The space without time, in which the soul determines upcoming life goals, lessons, and events. Here you can see whether you prearranged heart disease as a learning experience for this lifetime, and if you did, you have the opportunity to alter the plan.
- *The Gray Zone:* The place where space and time meet while the soul is exiting the White Zone and beginning its entry orbit into an awaiting body. Check here for cords or bindings, as people frequently attract interference on their way into an awaiting body.
- *The Red Zone:* The place where space and time meet while the soul, still lingering in the body, is just about to exit into the Black Zone. Many souls leave some of their life energy in the Red Zone. In the case of heart disease, you could have done so in order to help another soul or because of a tragic relationship. Return to this zone to see whether you must reclaim a part of your energy or break an attachment to another person.
- *The Black Zone:* The space without time just after death in which the soul pauses before deciding which way to go through the Planes of Light. At times, a part of the soul will linger here or get stuck. Heart conditions can indicate that you lost a part of yourself in the Black Zone in order to remain in a relationship. Release all attachments that you find.

Assistance on the Elemental Pathway

There are thousands of helpers you can call upon on the elemental pathway. This is a partial list; a longer one is available in my book *Advanced Chakra Healing*.

The Natural World Call upon the beings of the natural world to support your healing process.

- *Ancestors:* Can be summoned to clear genetic patterns or to release you from inherited patterns
- *Power animals and totems:* Can provide information, support, guidance, and healing
- *Plant spirits:* Can infuse your body with their energies for natural healing
- *Nature beings:* Can cleanse your environment or your body
- *Beings of earth, the stars, and planets:* Can support your healthy cells, provide guidance, and help you journey to other times and places

Elemental Beings Elemental beings can perform any number of services.

- *Water beings:* Can wash your system of poisons and decrease inflammation and plaque buildup.
- *Fire beings:* Can purge yeast, mold, fungus, viruses, and plaque. Can energize a sluggish system or stimulate a failing heart. Can sometimes burn away "wet" feelings, such as sadness. Can also eliminate toxins and waste products and get the lymph system flowing.
- *Metal beings:* Can provide boundaries and keep damaged organs from further injury.
- *Stone beings:* Can fortify and strengthen weak tissue, vessels, or valves to support tissue after surgery. Attach a stone being to your soul to keep your soul in your body during surgery or when undergoing a severe attack.

- *Wood beings:* Can restore balance and clarity. Use them to help repair an area after surgery and to tonify an organ that's been under stress.
- *Earth beings:* Can support the organic tissues of your body and help your body repair after surgery or after a stroke.
- *Air beings:* Can carry information, which is especially useful if you want to find the bottom-line cause of your heart problems or communicate with someone or something else. Use air beings to link your heart with other organs for entrainment, such as to "tell" them which frequency to use.
- *Light beings:* Can illuminate a bodily area or the underlying feeling or issue.
- *Ether beings:* Can infuse any cell, organ, or system with the correct spiritual energies or perception needed for healing. Can also deliver spiritual energies from the third layer of the energy egg to the physical body.
- *Star beings:* Can thoroughly cleanse and then reeducate any aspect of your system; especially helpful in rescuing and healing inner children.

Human Sources Don't forget your human helpers, living or dead! Here are ways to tap into them.

- Ask the Divine to find you the spirit of a well-known healer who is willing to help you.
- Ask the Divine to locate someone who has been healed of the type of heart disease you have.
- Ask for a guide from the past or the future who knows how to heal your type of heart condition.
- Look to the living! Friends, family, and professionals are there to help.

Aspects of the Self There are many inner aspects of the self that can help you heal.

- *The God self:* The self you would have been if raised with the Divine as your parents. Ask this self to provide input and healing, for it is already healthy.
- *The primal self:* This is a healthy part of your subconscious. Ask it to heal the fear- or shame-based parts of your subconscious and soul and connect you with divine grace. The primal self is motivated to help you survive and thrive.
- *The innocent child:* This self was never wounded by life experiences, so it is especially helpful in restoring the inner children who were injured.
- *The future self:* This self has already recovered from heart disease! Ask him or her to serve as a guide or to enter your body (perhaps through the etheric mirror) and bring you into your future healed state.
- *The master self:* In the Greater Reality, you have already perfected a certain set of gifts and skills. Ask that your master self step forward to assist you now.
- *The higher self:* This self understands fully the reasons you contracted a heart problem, but it has no pity. The higher self is an ideal healer, able to transmit healing energies straight from the Divine.

Many of these selves can help you assert the authority of your spirit's truth into your High Heart, and then invite the High Heart to manage the Middle and Lower Hearts.

Spiritual Sources There are thousands of spiritual sources that serve the Divine. They include angels, masters, avatars, saints, gurus, sorcerers of white magic, shamans, healers, and allies. I always ask the Divine to send the source most applicable for a certain need or time period.

chapter seven

Shift Healing on the Power Pathway

He who is able to conquer others is powerful; he who is able to conquer himself is more powerful.

—Lao-tzu, *Tao-te Ching*, chapter 33

Travel the power pathway under these conditions:

- You are clear about your primary disease chakra or the causes of your heart problem.
- You are interested in the supernatural and believe it can be commanded for personal benefit.
- You have shown some skill at working in the paranormal.
- You often work with the fifth, eighth, or eleventh chakra.

The Power Pathway: Breaking with Tradition

Without knowing it, most of us lose our lives following the path of tradition, succumbing to the pulls and pushes of everyday life, getting lost in the events that happen to us. We spend our lives pursuing what is in front of us, responding to stimulation without discovering that we are creators and directors.

The power pathway propels us into the position of authority. You cannot operate on the power pathway unless you are willing to seize your inner power and use it to establish life's parameters.

Heart Disease on the Power Pathway

On the power pathway, conquering heart disease is a matter of researching the forces and changing them if necessary. The power pathway looks like a system of spinning roles and cords, collectively called *spiritual energetic forces*. Healing is a matter of activating or deactivating these forces so you empower health and disempower disease. You have four main assignments on the power pathway:

1. Identify which spiritual energetic forces need to be switched on.
2. Identify which spiritual energetic forces need to be switched off.
3. Identify which forces need to be plugged in.
4. Identify which forces need to be pulled out.

The following tools will help you in your healing journey on the power pathway.

Energies on the Power Pathway

The primary energy bodies on the power pathway are the *seals*, which are attached to your chakras. There are many other power pathway energy bodies (described in detail in my book *Advanced Chakra Healing*), but I'm going to concentrate on the seals because they can lend you superhuman healing abilities.

The seals look like lenses that attach to each chakra on the front and the back. At birth, seals are usually "unset" or convex in relation to your body, leaving us little to no control over power energies. There is a design to this. We must earn the right to power because the appropriate use of forces demands skill and ethics.

Upon reaching emotional and spiritual maturation, we can more consciously and conscientiously set our seals. This act involves flipping the lenses connected to a chakra so the convex side faces the chakra center point. We can set one or more seals at a time, or all the seals at once. The concave bowl is then able to receive the spiritual energies of the universe, and the convex side focuses powers for personal use.

The seals transmit supernatural energies, which are available through commanding. These energies can blast away a blood clot or plaque, empower a weak heart valve, smooth an erratic heart-beat, relax tense muscle tissue, or create calm in a hypertensive moment. To access these forces, continue to work with the chakras on the elemental pathway, but after setting your seals, add or subtract forces to attach emphasis to your work. You can also read the center of a seal to examine it for spiritual energetic forces.

Here are descriptions of each seal and its primary relation-ship to heart disease.

Seal One: Brings spiritual matter into the physical body. You can rebuild the physical body after surgery or a stroke, support weak vessels, add power to a weak heart, or use the template from the etheric mirror described in the Special Insert and chapter 6 to create a healthy body.

Seal Two: Connects with feelings in forces. This seal will attract forces that can help you release repressed feelings or the feelings of others, as well as smooth the feelings creating heart disorders.

Seal Three: Works with consciousness waves instead of just thoughts. Consciousness waves are strong bands of thoughts that can implement immediate changes in beliefs and ideas. If your heart disorder involves emotional or mental strongholds, use this seal to align with the correct consciousness waves for a quick change of beliefs.

Seal Four: Focuses divine love. Can call on various spiritual energetic forces, such as the virtues and the overall energy of divine love, to bring relationships into balance. Almost all heart conditions involve erroneous assumptions about relationships. Use elemental healing symbols, numbers, shapes, or spin to establish the correct relationships among the self, other, and Divine, or among Low, Middle, and High Heart, for optimum work with this seal.

Seal Five: Uses auditory vibrations for immediate healing. Ask the Divine or higher guidance to speak or sing to you, and allow these healing messages to erase inaccurate ones or to educate you about love.

Seal Six: Activates visual information so it forms a template in the body. Picture your desired healed state. Now attach a force through this seal to the image of your desired healed state, and command the template into your body, thus willing your body to conform.

Seal Seven: Imprints consciousness and spiritual waves directly into the body. You can enforce a connection by willing a higher consciousness (especially through the High Heart or the pineal gland) into any organ or set of organs. Request help from a spiritual guide to work this way.

Seal Eight: Aligns the here and now with potentials from other planes and worlds. Here are several techniques for working with this seal.

- Focus on the God self, innocent child, or a healed self from the future, then align power forces with the physical body to integrate this self into the body.
- Summon energies or healers from other planes or dimensions and ask them to provide you with the spiritual energetic forces needed to heal from heart disease in this location.
- Bring a medication or technique "back" from the future to receive the cure now. Connect power pathway forces to

current healing supports, such as medication or herbs, to infuse the future effectiveness into the current healing support.

- Establish a generative or supportive force between your heart and the Divine's heart, and model your heart after the Divine's.

Seal Nine: Activates principles directly into the body. Ninth-chakra heart conditions mirror social problems. Go for a higher principle than one that allows self-sacrifice. How about focusing on "The Good of All," instead of "Giving for the Good of All"? Attach a degenerative force to the old philosophy and a generative force to the higher one.

Seal Ten: Aligns with vibrations of natural-world energies and beings. Intensify the healing power of an herb by applying a power pathway force. Eliminate toxins, clots, or plaque by attaching a generative power to a natural supplement or a degenerative nature-force to the block.

Seal Eleven: Through this seal, you can instantly vibrate a natural or supernatural energy to the millionth degree with a simple command. The challenge is to make sure you are calling forces through *resonance*, using vibration to discern which forces fit with particular goals.

Seal Twelve: Interfaces with all layers of the energy egg to draw in forces that alleviate our human concerns. Use this seal and applicable power forces to boost elemental healing through the first layer of the energy egg; make choices and seek new roads of health through the second layer of the energy egg; and connect with spiritual forces through the third layer of the energy egg.

There are two other energy bodies useful on the power pathway. The first is the etheric or Christ body, mentioned in the Special Insert and chapter 6. The second is the *Book of Life*. Similar to the Akashic Records (see pages 177 and page 228), this reservoir of knowledge contains everything you've ever done or experienced in the past, present, or potential future but only through the perspective of love. Later in this chapter, I offer exercises for working with both bodies on the power pathway.

Spiritual Energetic Forces on the Power Pathway Spiritual energetic forces are composed of multiple energies. These include quanta and such natural forces as magnetic, electrical, or electromagnetic forces, but they also stretch beyond the everyday to include pure consciousness and energies from other planes, planets, and dimensions. You will know which forces to use based on the principle of resonance, an important term in heart healing and one I discuss later in this chapter.

Here is a list of the basic spiritual energetic forces. For a more thorough explanation of each one, see my book *Advanced Chakra Healing.*

- *Spiritual forces:* These energies literally lock into your energy system or body and can remove or add energy. *Degenerative spiritual forces* take energy away, whereas *generative spiritual forces* add energy.
- *Powers:* The powers have the same labels as the elements: fire, water, earth, air, wood, metal, stone, ether, light, and star. These fundamental energies attach to the spiritual forces to provide a needed spin or quality to the connected spiritual force.
- *Virtues:* Virtues are energies holding ideals. They can shape your chakras and beliefs to conform to the concepts they represent. I usually establish virtues in the back of the chakras, through which they provide the greatest thrust.
- *Rays:* Rays are multidimensional energies that connect one chakra to another to help each attain ideal functioning. You can read more about them in my book *New Chakra Healing.*
- *Golden kundalini:* Golden kundalini is a process (described in the Special Insert) for raising the red serpent kundalini to

a spiritual level. This process magnifies the healing properties of your body and opens your spiritual gifts.

The Main Principle of Command: Resonance

You move energy on the power pathway through commanding. To *command* is to issue an order and expect that it will be carried out. The key to power pathway effectiveness is to understand what you are commanding and for what reason.

In heart healing, we seek to establish resonance inside the heart and between the heart and related organs. You want to align with energies that resonate with wholeness rather than brokenness.

To command for resonance, try the following.

Harmonizing for Health Exercise

1. If you're verbally adept, psychically listen to the tone of your spiritual harmonic, after conducting exercise five in the next section, to pinpoint your personal harmonic. Eliminate spiritual energetic forces that don't match your personal harmonic; use only those that do.

2. If you're visually gifted, psychically compare a spiritual energetic force with the coloration, hue, symbol, or other pictorial representation of your spiritual harmonic. Use forces that match or support your harmonic; relieve yourself of forces that do not.

3. If you're kinesthetic, sense, feel, smell, taste, or touch your spiritual harmonic in comparison with a spiritual energetic force. This will tell you which forces are good matches for you.

Safeguarding Your Power

Here are a few methods for safeguarding yourself.

1. *Check your body.* If you have misplaced or misused a spiritual energetic force, you will feel uncomfortable, uneasy, or ill. Ask the Divine to correct the situation instantly and to teach you what to do differently next time.

2. *Use a time lock.* You can establish time parameters for any energetic work. Command that a force attaches (or remains detached) only until the healing is accomplished.

3. *Align with your spiritual genetics.* Command that all spiritual energetic forces attune to your *spiritual genetics*, which are spiritual virtues encoded through your spirit into your body, especially into your High Heart. Those that don't align must simply detach or fall away.

4. *Utilize your etheric mirror.* Select only the spiritual energetic forces that match the template on your etheric mirror (see Special Insert).

5. *Remember your personal harmonic.* Check all forces for resonance using your personal harmonic. Command that your energy system accept only forces that attune to this harmonic and for only as long as the relationship is beneficial.

Special Power Pathway Techniques

Here are a few techniques that make best use of the power pathway.

Setting the Seals

A more thorough description of this process is offered in my book *Advanced Chakra Healing*. Here are the main steps:

Follow steps 1 and 2 in Five Steps for Safe Psychic Use provided in the Special Insert.

1. When you reach step 3, Conduct the goal, cleanse each chakra with breath or a golden-white light.
2. Ask the Divine to send a guide to help you set your seals.
3. Ask this guide to command each seal into its highest setting.
4. Visualize a cross of equal arms with a circle around it to lock the seal in place.
5. Ask the guide to instruct you in using the seals.

Heart Healing with the Golden Kundalini The golden kundalini can help you access your serpent or red kundalini and bolster your basic life energy. Ask the Divine to start the process in love and faith. (For a complete description of how to initiate your golden kundalini, see my book *Advanced Chakra Healing*.)

Keying into Your Spiritual Harmonic Harmonics represent your major spiritual truths, such as honesty, love, truth, or caring. These truths compose your *spiritual genetics*, chromosome-like structures of light that form your true self. Heart disease would clear immediately if you enacted all your spiritual genes in your body. Working with your spiritual harmonic assists you in this integration process.

You may have more than one key harmonic or spiritual attribute, but usually there is a primary one. There are exercises for identifying your key personal harmonic in my book *Advanced Chakra Healing*; for a shortcut, think of the happiest moment in your life, then decide which spiritual truth best reflects the reason that you were so happy. The truths that surface are related to your harmonic.

Reading the Book of Life for Heart Healing

To summon the Book, command its presence, ask for a guide to assist you, or visualize the Book of Life that is your own and turn its pages to find your answers. Once you have what you are looking for, you can do any of the following.

Reading the Past Travel backward in time to find the reason you now have heart disease, using the Regression Exercise in the Special Insert. Then use the Forgiveness Exercise in the insert to release yourself from past "mistakes." Seen through the lens of love, of course, you will learn that you have never made a mistake!

Reading the Present Journey through the Book of Life to find the self who has the secrets to healing your heart. To read the present, use the exercises in the Special Insert, including Find Your Fragments and Heal Yourself, the exercises listed under Moving Through Time for Information and Healing, and the steps provided for energy mapping and diagnosis. Gather the energy, knowledge, wisdom, cure, healing substance, or energy from this self and call forth a strong generative spiritual force to bring it into your body.

Reading the Future There is a future self who is healed of heart disease. Use the Futuring Exercise in the Special Insert to travel through the Book of Life to find your future self and discuss the healing path. Bring this knowledge or healing energy back with you. Add spiritual energetic forces to assist with the changes in your body.

Transmission through the Etheric Mirror Work with your primary disease chakra or your heart. Call forth the generative spiritual force of connection, which will appear as a band of light. Connect the chakra or seal with the etheric mirror and command that the codes needed to create healing and resonance transfer from that energy body into your physical body. Intensify this process using spiritual energetic forces that harmonize with your own spirit.

Summoning Authority against Interference Often, heart disease on the power pathway can be diagnosed as interference: ideas, feelings, entities, cords, curses, or other energies that disrupt your natural resonance. This section will show you how to combat these interferences wisely and safely.

First, determine what is causing the disruption in your primary chakra site, its affiliate organ, or your heart. Second, ask the Divine to isolate that interruptive energy. Now do one of the following:

- *Force with spiritual forces:* Consider two different spiritual forces. Attach one to the "good guy," your internal organ or chakra, and the other to the "bad guy," the intruder. Now set these spiritual forces against each other by establishing them in opposing spins, shapes, tones, colors, and speeds.
- *Disempower with powers:* Raw powers can be used very effectively in opposition. Select two opposing powers, such as fire and water, and attach one to the intruder and one to your internal organ or chakra. Connect a generative spiritual force to yourself and a degenerative spiritual force to the intruder. This will compel the enemy out of your body.
- *By virtue of virtues:* As with the other exercises, select two virtues that are different enough to seem contrary. Attach one to the intruder and one to your internal organ or chakra, and again, increase their potency with spiritual forces or powers. The relationship will terminate altogether.

Helpers on the Power Pathway

Here is an introduction to a few of the beings available on the power pathway. A more detailed description of these beings is available in my book *Advanced Chakra Healing*.

- *Angels:* Teams of angels work together toward a specific helpful objective, such as healing, cleanup, or restoration. They can guide you in the correct forces with which to work, show you pictures in the seals, and help you change forces. The angels of death can convey abilities that you "left on the other side" before you were born.
- *Entity forms:* These are entities that can transform energies from one form to another. You can also request the services

of an entity form that has developed the skill of transformation. You might employ the services of a being capable of shifting plaque to a benign element, for instance, to rid yourself from the long-term side effects of plaque buildup.

- *The shining ones:* These bring spiritual energies into the physical plane. Ask them to deliver energies to sustain your healthy cells or to create resonance.
- *The powers:* The powers are beings that send material energies into spiritual dimensions. Use them to spirit away intruders, interference, and physical problems, such as clots or plaque.
- *Archetypes:* These help you model love, the key to healing heart disease.
- *Muses:* Muses can generate your own spiritual harmonic, which you can use to hold the tones of the spiritual energetic forces.
- *The ideals:* These are beings that assist in the correct placement and ordering of the virtues needed to support a healthy body.
- *The virtues:* These are entities that command the properties of divine love, the greatest healing energy of all.
- *The forces:* These are beings that stand ready to help you select, discard, or choose spiritual forces.
- *Masters and avatars:* These beings can help you make decisions and work clearly with the power pathway energies.

chapter eight

Shift Healing on the Imagination Pathway

*I don't mean another planet, you know; they're part of our world
and you could get to them if you went far enough—but a really Other
World—another Nature—another universe—somewhere you would
never reach even if you traveled through the space of this universe for
ever and ever—a world that could be reached only by Magic—well!*
—C.S. Lewis, *The Magician's Nephew*†

Travel the imagination pathway under these conditions:

- You can imagine a future different than one that includes heart disease.

- You are willing to accept responsibility for having and therefore changing your heart problem.

- You have previously used your imagination when creating your reality.

- You believe that there are many possible futures, not just one.

- You have shamanic interests and abilities.

- You seek to complement your work on another pathway with magical means.

- You often use your sixth, eighth, or tenth chakra.

†Lewis, C.S., *The Chronicls of Narnia. The Original Novels. The Magician's Nephew*
(New York: Harper Trophy, 2002), p.21.

The Imagination Pathway:
The Magic of Imagination

One night, a star fell to earth. She was shocked to find herself alone and cold, instead of hanging in the dark, warm sky. Thought Little Star, I will be all right. I'll just shine really bright and people will notice and take care of me.

But that's not what happened. When people look to the sky, they expect to see the sky full of blazing lights. When they look at their feet, they think to see nothing—and so nothing is what they see. And so Little Star was doomed to lie unseen, sad and alone on the earth. Her light dwindled, and she almost stopped being at all, when one day, a little boy stumbled on her.

"Look, Mom!" said the little boy. "A star!"

The mother couldn't see the star. Neither could the boy's father. All they could see was a cold, ugly stone. Frustrated, they told their son to stop pretending. "You will teach your sister bad manners," they said. Weren't they appalled when the little sister—and the dog, as well—could see Little Star?

Because someone could see her, Little Star began to believe in her own power again. Believing in herself, she grew strong and bold, and one evening, she was able to reach upward with one of her long arms and pull herself back into the sky! That is where she hangs today, looking over the little boy and his sister and their dog.

This story illustrates the power of the imagination. If you believe in something, you are most of the way to making it real. The little boy believed he had found a star, even though the rock looked more like a lump of coal than a shiny sky diamond. The boy's belief enabled the fallen star to return to her place in the heavens as a real star. Why was the little boy able to see a star in a rock, when no one else could? He didn't know he wasn't supposed to!

Do you know that you can heal from heart disease? Has a doctor, friend, book, statistic, or inner fear told you you couldn't? Do you believe that? Then it's time to work on the imagination pathway for two reasons: first, to start believing in your own heart and its power to heal, and second, to break with the tradition of illness and begin the life you want to lead.

Heart Disease on the Imagination Pathway

There is a correlation between quantum physics, heart disease, and your imagination. As discussed in chapter 2, quantum physics has revealed that there are many different types of particles that compose physical reality and that these particles don't have to follow human logic when deciding how to behave.

Subatomic particles can pretty much go anywhere and in any time and a part of you that can track and even control the movement of these bits of matter. That part of you is your imagination!

By means of intuition, your imagination is able to perceive the placement, composition, and purposes of the particles that make up matter, the quanta of the universe. If you have a heart condition, it's because some of the particles making up your heart aren't supporting your health. Change the quanta, change your health.

You can imagine yourself well—but just seeing something doesn't make it so. You have to *motivate* the quanta to form a new reality before the new reality can *manifest*.

Something motivated your body to create a heart problem. That something could be physical in orientation, such as a virus or a genetic defect. The motivation could be emotional, such as repressed anger, or mental, such as the belief that you don't deserve love. It could even be spiritual, as in the religious idea that if you've been bad, God will punish you with a disease. *If something motivated you to become ill, something else can motivate you to become well.*

Your imagination is the tool that can show you the possibility of wellness. Envisioning what you want is the first step in healing on the imagination pathway. To make the shift from illness to health, you must decide to exchange the current reality for a new one. Then you must live as if the new reality were not only possible but already in existence.

Walking into the Imagination

Each chakra houses a lens that looks like a mirror. On one side of the mirror lies the world as you know it. Here are the quanta supportive of heart disease. On the other side of the mirror is an entirely different universe, called the antiworld. Here are all the different possible worlds that could be, if we just decided to make them real.

The heart is especially empowered to make the decisions necessary to change your reality because it is the center of the energetic system. The heart is uniquely composed of equal amounts of tachyon (fast) and quark (slow) particles and waves.

What you think,

you can become.

What you feel, you

can manifest.

What you want,

you can have.

The heart as the giving and receiving organ in your body will accept as much goodness as you allow yourself to have. Decide what you want, and hold it as your heart's desire. Within you are all the powers necessary to open to the assistance and love necessary to change reality.

The following tools will help you in your journey on the imagination pathway.

Energies on the Imagination Pathway

You won't find energy bodies on the imagination pathway. Instead of looking for structure, spend your time tracking the dance of the quanta. Look for negative, positive, and neutral energies, and fast- and slow-moving information. To eliminate heart disease, the energies you need are in the antiworld, on the other side of the *imagination mirror*. You can work with the imagination mirror by checking for three components.

1. A white side, upon which you see what is currently "true"
2. A black side, which reveals what exists in other worlds or dimensions
3. An empty, neutral space in the middle, from which you can make diagnoses and exchange energies between worlds

To use this mirror you must use your *imagination*—the part of your mind that can conjure images, pictures, and knowing. When working on the imagination pathway, you'll be standing in your shaman self, the part of you that links and walks within all worlds. Through the imagination pathway, your shamanic self can accomplish the following.

· Identify what's going on here and now
· See into a different spacetime or antiworld to see what is possible
· Try on or test different life choices
· Neutralize a bad situation
· Exchange energies between the worlds
· Lock new changes into place

Two Useful Energy Tools

I strongly recommend becoming familiar with two useful energy tools on the imagination pathway. The first is your Akashic Records, which I described in the Special Insert and chapter 6. The second energy tool involves working through the second layer of the energy egg, also described in the Special Insert. This layer relates to the unconscious; it contains all the ideas and possibilities hidden there. If you can perceive new choices in the second layer of your energy egg and accept them, your unconscious can lock them in place.

Visualize the second layer of the energy egg in the imagination mirror. It looks like a milky-white dream space, in which you can perceive images, ideas, and possibilities. Once you have chosen one of the possibilities you find in this layer, connect it to the third layer of the energy egg and allow the Divine to bring the entire possibility into your being.

Energy Symbology and Vibration

As with all other pathways, you are working vibrationally on the imagination pathway. One of the easiest ways to work with the quanta is to use energy symbols and techniques to establish form. When you enforce a symbol with decisiveness, the quanta must do what you want.

In the imagination mirror, you can diagnose whether your heart or a disease-related chakra is infested with too many negative or positive qualities, or whether these or the neutral quanta are improperly programmed. As on the other pathways, negative elements will be dark and held in boxy rather than circular shapes, and fit most of the other criteria spelled out in chapter 4. Positive elements will be light-colored, spinning forward, and holding more circular shapes. If neutral quanta are inappropriately programmed, they won't look like their normal, shiny, rose or white selves; they will be discolored, dull, and murky.

The imagination mirror provides an additional diagnostic step in that you can check for direction and destination of the quanta. Which way are the energies spinning? Negative energies spin in reverse, positive spiral forward, and neutral remain still. The key is to track how these energies are spinning or what they are affecting.

On the imagination pathway, you can check for and work with the same concepts as the elemental pathway: spin, coloration, symbology, tones, cords and other connections, and links to other planes, dimensions, and zones. You can experiment before you lock a change into place. Even if you make a mistake, you can undo it!

Special Imagination Pathway Techniques

Here are some techniques specific to the imagination pathway:

- *Locking in a change:* Lock imagination pathway changes into the imagination mirror, so that the energies transferred from one side of reality don't slip back. Any symbol, shape, number, or tone will work, as will prayer or intention. I also use a cross with equal arms within a circle because of its universal power.

- *Diagnosing from this side of reality:* Place yourself in the chakra involved in your heart condition. Look at the mirror on this side of reality to see the cause of your heart disease.

- *Healing from the other side of reality:* Center yourself in the chakra involved in the heart condition. Jump through the mirror, into the antiworld of this chakra. What would your life look like from this point of view? The image holds the energies needed to be healthy in this time and space. Gather the image and its energies, and leap back into the this-world side of the mirror. Paint the mirror with your new portrait, and ask the Divine to send the old life into the antiworld. Then ask the Divine to infuse your new life with power, so your empowered life becomes more and more real each day.

- *Diagnosing and healing through the center of the mirror:* There is an empty space in the center of the mirror. Stand here and you can look at both sides of your imagination reality, then use them for diagnosing and healing.

- *Commanding forces through the center of the mirror:* The center of an imagination mirror is a place of authority. Here, you can access the powers and forces of the power pathway to create masterful change. Command your desires from this center place and watch as the energies shift. Lock in your changes.

- *Walking through the mirror:* Bring your awareness into your primary disease chakra. Feel your feelings in regard to having heart disease. Now gather these energies and picture a large black door in the imagination mirror. Leap through this door into the realm that is free of heart problems. Exchange the healthy energies for the unhealthy ones, and look at the imagination door. You'll notice it has become white. When you walk back into "real reality," this white door will filter all energies associated with heart disease. Return to this world, and lock in your changes with a symbol.

- *Cipher healing:* Center in your primary disease chakra, look through the this-world mirror, and ask to see the symbol or shape anchoring the heart disease in this world. To understand this symbol better, work with the symbol meanings in the Special Insert or perform a regression or projection using the Special Insert exercises. After comprehending the reasons for your condition, decide whether you are willing to learn a different way. If so, transfer healing energies (these can be in symbol form) from the antiworld and release disease energies from this world.

- *Casing the Akashic Records:* Within the primary disease chakra, look at the this-world mirror and ask to see your Akashic Records. Now ask to review the situation that led to your condition; it may play like a movie or filmstrip. The Akashic Records can reveal situations pertaining to this or past lives. Next, flip the mirror so you can see the antidote or cure. Exchange your old story for a new one, and lock in the solution.

- *Embracing the shadow:* Within the primary disease chakra, peer into the this-world mirror and ask to see your heart condition. Do you see a shadowy energy around the images? This is the Shadow Record; it contains information about the hidden causes of your heart problems, especially those related to mistakes or regrets. Examine the shadows until you gain information about errors leading to the heart problem, then ask whether you are willing to forgive yourself. Transfer forgiveness into this side of reality, and allow the forgiveness to heal you.

- *Going for second is best:* Access the second layer of the energy egg by journeying or consciously traveling through the imagination layer into the realm of possibilities. Accept the desired energies and bring them into this world through the mirror, knowing that what you've brought in will displace the old reality. Lock these changes into place.

Helpers on the Imagination Pathway

Thousands of helpers are available to your shaman self on the imagination pathway. Many of these beings or energies are described in the Special Insert and in my book *Advanced Chakra Healing*; others can be reached through your imagination!

Before linking with the invisible, check first to see whether you are attached to any animate or inanimate sources that are supporting your heart condition.

A SPECIAL BULLETIN ON EVIL When working with heart disease, I always check for the effects or presence of evil. Evil describes beings and energies that seek to annul life. Rather than support consciousness, evil upholds anticonsciousness. Many heart problems stem from the effects and fears of evil. Fear will disrupt the proper function of any organ that houses it. The Divine is stronger than any force of evil. Evil can work only through trickery.

Evil forces usually work by convincing their prey to give away their power, which evil forces then use to create delusions and mirages that make themselves seem powerful. Conquer evil by asking the Divine to help you perceive an evil force for what it really is.

Turn all evils over to God, and ask for divine healing from the affects of being associated with evil. And remember, being affected by evil isn't the same as actually being evil yourself.

chapter nine

Shift Healing on the Divine Pathway

When I write of hunger, I am really writing about love and the
hunger for it, and warmth and the love of it that is all one.
  —M.F.K. Fisher, *The Gastronomical Me*†

T̲ravel the divine pathway under these conditions:

· You are concerned about your chances for survival.

· You are convinced that your heart condition is related to issues about love.

· You believe in the power of the Divine.

· You want to complement your work on another pathway with spiritual truth.

· You are willing to accept a miracle.

· You rely frequently on your third, seventh, or ninth chakra.

The Divine Pathway: Healing through Love

What if you could wake up and be well?

If there is a goal on the divine pathway, it is to awaken. Most of us live in slumber. If our parents didn't know their true value,

†Fisher, M.F.K., *The Gastronomical Me* (New York: North Point Press, 1989).

KEYS TO THE KINGDOM *Petitioning* is the main healing vehicle on the divine pathway. Petitioning is a form of prayer, quite simply communicating in a heartfelt way with the Divine. *Intercessory prayer* is making a request for someone else. *Meditation* involves turning your will and mind over to the Divine so that God prays for you. *Contemplation* is basking in the presence of the Divine. These are all communication methods on the divine pathway.

You can petition for anything, anytime, anyplace, anyhow, anywhere, and for anyone. On the divine pathway, you can actually direct your prayers to just about anyone, too, for everything and everyone is unified. Petition a cloud for water, and the cloud's consciousness will somehow get your request to a cistern or a water well company. Petition God, and God will send your dispatch to the closest angel, animal, tree, mailman—whatever or whomever is in the position to best fulfill the need. The deciding factor will never be a "what" or a "who"; it will be the presence of love in your heart.

we don't know our own. And if we live without full recognition of love, we are half asleep.

As a result of this half-sleep state, we don't allow ourselves to experience fully the breadth and depth of life, the cut and touch of relationship, the tears and joys of the everyday. We don't open to others' appreciation or needs. We don't see the Divine in every flower petal or gust of wind; we block our feelings and sensations so as to avoid facing our fears, beliefs that we are unlovable or not good enough. Operating on harmful beliefs, our inner heart eventually closes down, and so does our physical heart.

I believe that almost everyone on this planet has a heart condition, for almost no one allows the flow of unconditional love. Healing on the divine pathway occurs the moment you are willing to receive and give unconditional love. This state is called *wakefulness*. To awaken is to embrace the truth of love. The process of owning this truth is called *illumination*.

Illumination comes slowly. Part of the illumination process is acknowledging your imperfection and shadows, your unkindness and cruelty, the stuff that composes your "dark self." The dark self lives in the heart, for the heart is where we hide all our dangerous secrets. If you can see the dark self through the lens of love rather than the judgments of the world, however, you will find that it isn't such a very bad self; rather, the dark self is the sum total of all your misunderstandings about love. As you shine the light of love on the dark self, you will discover that dark isn't merely the absence of light; it is the container of light yet unseen.

Inevitably, healing on the divine pathway involves giving up the idea of personal perfection. The dark self stays secreted because it thinks that it is bad to be imperfect. The truth is that as a human, you will always have devious desires. You will err and make mistakes. You will be harmed and will hurt others. *Achieving wakefulness and the ensuing healing has nothing to do with being perfect.* To illuminate into wakefulness is to blend the human and the divine, the imperfect and the perfect, the errors with the achieved; to love and to live; to live with love.

How does love actually heal on the divine pathway? Through the perspective of the divine pathway, all illness, disease, and problems are cries for love. The dark self conducts and displays disease to get attention and healing. Meet the need for love through a method different than illness, and the illness can disappear. Illuminate the real need, and all needs are met, including that of physical healing.

As long as you can love, you can heal your heart.

The Heart on the Divine Pathway

What needs to be stitched, eliminated, or created is first accomplished in the space of spirit. And this healing is done through recognizing that the healing is finished before it has begun.

The heart, in comparison with other organs, is particularly responsive to prayer and other means of concentrated healing because the heart lies in the center of the human energy system. The heart blends the physical powers of the lower energy centers with the spiritual truths of the upper energy centers. By inviting the awakening of our hearts, we often allow the healing of our hearts. Work with any or all of the chakras involved with your heart problem and the healing energies will be translated into the physical heart.

On the divine pathway, you face your personal issues and work on archetypal issues, such as those presented in what I call the "bowls of existence." Within each chakra lies a pool of dark energies that must be transformed or transcended to achieve spiritual healing and therefore physical health. These bowls or pools represent universal challenges, such as the challenge of evil or death. The exercises in this section are fashioned to help you summon the courage and strength to look into the bowls of darkness and find your light.

The following tools will help you as journey on the divine pathway.

Energies on the Divine Pathway

Energy bodies unique to the divine pathway include:

- *Incandescent bodies:* These include the *bodies of the eternal and the infinite*, which allow you to break free of the space-time continuum.
- *Seven bowls of existence:* These hold humanity's greatest challenges.
- *Seven channels of light:* These are the seven primary chakras, each representing a divine truth. I have added another five channels to assist with the main chakras.
- *Twelve spiritual gates:* These are the evolved twelve auric bands.
- *Energy egg:* This is described in the Special Insert.

These energy bodies are described in detail in my book *Advanced Chakra Healing*. Following are ways to employ the divine energy bodies for healing the heart.

The Chakras and the Bowls

It's helpful to pinpoint which chakra contains the root of your heart disease; the issue is reflected in the bowl of this chakra. If you are not certain, work with the heart chakra itself.

On the divine pathway, petitioning will allow your chakras to transform into channels of light, forces for miraculous change. You can use the following chart to determine the need you must address in order to heal the issue facing you. The bowls associated with chakra eight through twelve are best understood in relation to spiritual gates, which are discussed next.

Divine Needs and Corresponding Chakra

Chakra/ Channel of Light	Need Shown by the Condition	Bowl: The Challenge Posed by the Condition
One	Self-definition, being "I"	Evil
Two	Being yourself	Death
Three	Self-determination	Judgment
Four	Connection through love	Power
Five	Communication through love	Suffering
Six	Evolution of self	False miracles
Seven	Change through purpose	Endings
Eight	Undoing what shouldn't have been	(See Spiritual Gates)
Nine	Being hopeful	(See Spiritual Gates)
Ten	Accepting what is now	(See Spiritual Gates)
Eleven	Accepting grace	(See Spiritual Gates)
Twelve	Truth of grace	(See Spiritual Gates)

The Spiritual Gates The auric bands transform into the twelve spiritual gates on the divine pathway. The chakras help you informationally, but the gates hold your desired changes in place. Heart problems always involve boundary issues related to love, specifically related to giving and receiving. You can give away love or refuse to accept it, take it in but neglect to send it, love others but not yourself, or love the Divine but not others. There are dozens of permutations, and any can result in heart disease. Miracles can occur when you study the auric bands for the source of boundary issues; address the spiritual issues involved on the divine pathway; and translate the changes into one, several, or all bands. When an auric band is inspired correctly, it transforms immediately into a spiritual gate and physical changes follow.

Each of the twelve spiritual gates relates to a specific chakra. Here is a synopsis of the meaning of each spiritual gate.

The Twelve Spiritual Gates

Gate (Auric Field)	Meaning
Gate One	Provides vital source of energy
Gate Two	Illuminates feelings to express spirit
Gate Three	Conveys highest truths
Gate Four	Awakens divine love
Gate Five	Provides full knowing
Gate Six	Reveals deepest truths
Gate Seven	Accesses Greater Consciousness
Gate Eight	Anchors the present
Gate Nine	Supports imperfection with compassion
Gate Ten	Reveals Greater Consciousness through nature
Gate Eleven	Creates perfection from imperfection
Gate Twelve	Accesses divine grace within self

Refer to my book *Advanced Chakra Healing* for a more detailed description of the gates and to learn how to incorporate the gates into your healing. I have also included an exercise in this chapter, called Healing through the Gates, in the section Special Divine Pathway Techniques. On the divine pathway, you will work with both the chakra and its associated gate for the first seven chakras (channels of light); beyond the seventh chakra, you will work with the auric band/gate.

The Energy Egg On the divine pathway, working with the third layer of the energy egg is powerful, because the third layer links with the outer layer of the twelfth chakra and auric band, and it opens the door to the spiritual realms that lie outside of the physical universe. Through this third layer, you can call energies that have never been seen or experienced, or form new healing forces at will. This becomes a *spiritual truth*, an idea that unifies two contrasting ideas. Heart healing often involves those "eureka!" moments, in which we see how two divergent concepts, conflicting events, or rival needs are one and the same. I have included an exercise in this chapter, called Egg-stra Effects, Healing through the Third Layer, in the section Special Divine Pathway Techniques.

Radiant Kundalini Radiant kundalini is another powerful healing tool on the divine pathway. Within each and every part of your body lives a pulsing center, beating in time with the heart of God. Connect to the rhythm of this luminescent white kundalini, and you can empower your heart and circulatory system with the energy of the Divine. A special technique for using this kundalini for heart disease healing is described in the upcoming section, Special Divine Pathway Techniques.

Petitioning for a Purpose: The Key to Divine Healing

Are you ready to create physical changes through the divine pathway? Read the sidebar, Keys to the Kingdom, at the beginning of this chapter. Remember that petitioning is to make a request of the Divine. Send out your prayers—the people, forces, or helpers in the best position to serve will receive them. Ask for what you think you need, and you will receive what you really need. Seek healing, and the request shall be answered in the way and time that is of the highest good. Here are a few suggestions:

- Ask the Divine to create your petition for you.
- Ask the Divine to grant your petition according to divine will.

- Ask to be a true vehicle for unconditional love, and the love pouring through you shall also heal you.

The Divine wants you to be happy. Surrender to divine will and you will receive what you need to become happier.

Special Divine Pathway Techniques

Here are a few techniques for healing heart disease on the divine pathway.

From Chakras to Channels of Light Healing occurs quickly after you transform a chakra into a channel of light, because you are then able to direct spiritual energies into the body for physical results. Ask the Divine to transform your primary disease chakra, your heart chakra, or all your chakras while you are sleeping. Upon waking, center your thoughts in the middle of the most appropriate chakra, and ask the Divine to send you the spiritual truth that will provide physical healing to your body. Embrace this truth. Ask how you can live and express this during the day, so as to lock this truth into your body and mind. If you feel called to do so, re-create this exercise every morning. Now you are becoming a channel of light!

Radiation through Radiating To conduct healing through the radiant kundalini, center your attention in the middle of the primary disease chakra or your heart chakra. Ask the Divine to bring through the spiritual truths and energies needed to transform your body through the power of unconditional love. Acknowledge that you are receiving a full healing.

Egg-stra Effects, Healing through the Third Layer The power of the third layer of the energy egg is ultimately the power of faith. Center yourself in your heart and ask to stand in the full energy of faith. Do you feel lacking? Ask the Divine to share its faith in you with you. As you open to this inflow of support, petition the Divine to open your heart channel to the third layer of your energy egg. What spiritual truths need to flow into your body to release you from your heart condition? Simply allow the Divine or your own higher self to select the energies required, or formulate them on the spot.

Loving Your Heart If your heart is presenting you with a condition, it is only because it seeks a deeper form of understanding and love. Ask your heart, "In what ways am I not full of love?" Now, literally talk to your heart, asking what it needs in terms of behavior, attitudes, or changes in belief or feelings to allow divine healing. Listen and act on its response.

Allowing Miracles Brain research has shown that emotions play a critical role in rational decision making. Emotions are also critical in allowing miracles. It's easier to allow healing when we hold emotions that are peaceful, hopeful, and grateful. Simply ask the Divine to replace worries and self-destructive emotions with more optimistic and life-enhancing ones.

Another approach for inviting miracles is to challenge societal thinking, which states that miracles are irrational. Popular culture defines the miraculous as unexplained or extraordinary phenomenon. This characterization presents spiritual healing as somewhat irrational. Challenge this rationale with the question "Why would God want me to be unhappy and sick?"

Helpers on the Divine Pathway

Everything and everyone in this and all other worlds wants to help you heal. Petition the Divine, and the Divine will appoint the helper that will best speed you toward wellness and peace. You can also ask for special guides, which might include angels, as well as the following:

- *Aspects of the self*, such as your innocent child, who can heal your inner children; your God self, who can parent you; your future self, who is already healed; and your master self, who already has the tools to clear your heart problems

- *Masters and avatars* that can share specific knowledge with you about your healing
- *Guardians* of spiritual realms present and beyond the third layer of the energy egg
- *Religious figures*, such as saints and ancestors, can help you merge your divine and human selves

chapter ten

The Heart of Faith

Faith is to believe what you do not see; the reward
of this faith is to see what you believe.

—St. Augustine

Faith on the Pathways

A lot of people ask me whether their hearts will heal if they lack faith: faith in God, in healing, in themselves, in their surgeons. When we're sick, the list of people, places, and energies we think we must believe in can seem endless.

There is really one type of faith that matters, and that is a faith in the power of love.

One of my favorite healing stories is about Mahatma Gandhi, who was a strict vegetarian and pacifist. Gandhi didn't believe in Western medicine, including medication and surgery, which he found intrusive. Rather, he used diet, exercise, and prayer when he was sick.

One evening, Gandhi was stricken with acute appendicitis and was taken to Colonel Maddock, a British surgeon general. Maddock recommended surgery. A day later, Gandhi affirmed the choice, writing a statement claiming full confidence in Maddock and the surgery. Gandhi's life was saved, despite the fact that he shifted outside of his comfort zone and agreed to an operation.[1]

I believe the reason Gandhi was healed of appendicitis through a means not typically believable to him can be explained through the Four Pathways philosophy. Most of the time, Gandhi lived on the divine pathway. Without perceiving it, however, he fully dwelled on the elemental and all the other pathways. Thanks to appendicitis, Gandhi was forced to connect with his elemental self, which was fully ready to believe in conventional medicine. Whether or not his everyday, spiritual self believed in the elemental pathway modalities such as drugs and surgery, Gandhi's elemental self already had the necessary faith. At some level, Gandhi realized that the *instrument* of his healing might be elemental, but the *power* that could induce the healing was faith.

And what was the source of this power? He lived a life of love, and he daily exhibited faith in the power of love. To encompass a perspective different from his own, Gandhi simply expanded his faith in love a little wider, to embrace faith in his surgeon and the surgery. What Gandhi did, we can all do.

The Power of Faith

Jesus frequently bears witness to the power of faith. "Truly, I say to you, if you have faith and never doubt ... even if you say to this mountain, 'Be taken up and cast into the sea,' it will be done."[2] I don't see many mountains moving in my house, much less children when I suggest it's time to do homework or clean a bedroom! Nonetheless, I don't question my faith in the power of love.

What is this power of faith, and how do we apply it to pathway healing? Faith is built into pathway healing because it is innate to your heart. We are all equipped with the faith needed to love and be loved, to heal and be healed, and this is because we already live fully within the Greater Reality.

Belief is a strong element in faith, but we don't necessarily have to believe something to be true to effect change. What if we simply have faith that we are filled with faith? If we accept that the Greater Reality, the only true reality, is based on love, we need only have faith in the power of love, and healing will simply occur, on whatever pathway and in whatever time is most loving for ourselves.

I propose that this faith in love is the basis of all healing, especially pathway healing. It is the key to accessing the chakras, shifting energies for healing, and accepting the grace that has been present all along. To be truly wakeful, to be illuminated, is nothing more—or less—than knowing that God so loves us, that God believes in us! The faith we need lies within our hearts, the very organ that seems to now challenge our survival.

Underneath the presenting issue is the solution to the problem. Have faith that love dwells within, and you have all the faith necessary to heal. Find your heart, and you hold the power to heal.

Conclusion:
Awakening Love
through the Chakras

I have faith in pathway healing because I have seen it work.

I have held hands with a little girl who, scared to death, was blue from lack of oxygen. We prayed, and she healed, and her cheeks are now as rosy as her future.

I have discussed a diagnosis with a well-known musician, asking her to see a doctor for a particular test. She called back. A rare disease did exist in her body. After treatment, the angina and coronary artery blockage disappeared. The elemental treatment has given her a future, a new life.

I have suggested to a young man that he dig deep inside and begin to use his natural powers. This single idea encouraged him to go to his heart and substitute one spiritual force for another. His ventricular fibrillations ceased from that point forward.

The power to heal lies within every part of our body and self, but particularly within and because of our hearts. We have only to know that we are loved to have enough faith to accept the gifts of love: joy, happiness, and healing.

Pathway Reading Lists

Part I

Begley, Sharon, *The Hand of God*, Philadelphia: Templeton Foundation Press, 1999.

Benson, Herbert, M.D., *Timeless Healing*, New York: Scribner, 1997.

Braden, Gregg, *The God Code*, Carlsbad, CA: Hay House, 2004.

Challem, Jack, *The Inflammation Syndrome*, Hoboken, New Jersey: John Wiley & Sons, 2003.

Dale, Cyndi, *New Chakra Healing*, St. Paul, MN: Llewellyn Publications, 1998.

Dossey, Larry, M.D., *Reinventing Medicine*, San Francisco: HarperSanFrancisco: 1999.

Gerber, Richard, M.D., *Vibrational Medicine*, Rochester, VT: Bear & Company, 2001.

Greene, Brian, *The Fabric of the Cosmos*, New York: Vintage Books, 2004.

Hawking, Stephen, Ph.D., *The Universe in a Nutshell*, New York: Bantam Books, 2001.

Hubbard, Barbara Marx, *Conscious Evolution*, Novato, CA: New World Library, 1998.

Hunt, Valerie, *Infinite Mind*, Malibu, CA: Malibu Publishing, 1996.

McCartney, Francesca, Ph.D., *Body of Health: The New Science of Intuition Medicine for Energy & Balance*, Novato, CA: Nataraj Publishing, 2005.

Orloff, Judith, M.D., *Second Sight*, New York: Warner Books, 1997.

Oschman, James L., *Energy Medicine*, Philadelphia, PA: Churchill Livingstone, 2000.

Pearsall, Paul, M.D., *The Heart's Code*, New York: Broadway, 1999.

Rippe, James M., M.D., *Heart Disease for Dummies*, Hoboken, NJ: Wiley Publishing, 2004.

Ross, Julia, M.A., *The Diet Cure*, New York: Penguin Books, 1999.

Sheldrake, Rupert, *A New Science of Life*, Rochester, VT: Park Street Press, 1995.

Siegel, Bernie, S., *Love, Medicine & Miracles*, New York: Harper & Row, Publishers, Inc., 1986.

Simpson, Liz, *The Book of Chakra Healing*, London: Gaia Books Limited, 1999.

Talbot, Michael, *The Holographic Universe*, New York: HarperCollins Publishers, 1991.

Weil, Andrew, M.D., *Health and Healing*, New York: Houghton Mifflin Co., 1998.

Wolf, Fred Alan, Ph.D., *Taking the Quantum Leap*, New York: Harper & Row Publishers, 1981.

Zukav, Gary, *The Seat of the Soul*, New York: Simon & Schuster, 1989.

Additional Resources:

Publications from the HeartMath Research Center, Institute of HeartMath, www.heartmath.org.

Part II

Elemental

Amen, Daniel, M.D., *Change Your Brain, Change Your Life*, New York: Three Rivers Press, 1998.

Balch, James F., M.D., and Stengler, Mark, N.D., *Prescription for Natural Cures*, New York: John Wiley & Sons, 2004.

Braverman, Debra, M.D., *Heal Your Heart with EECP*, Berkeley, CA: Celestial Arts, 2005.

Brennan, Barbara Ann, *Hands of Light*, New York: Bantam, 1988.

Burns, David D., M.D., *The Feeling Good Handbook*, New York: Plume, The Penguin Group, 1999.

Carper, Jean, *The Miracle Heart: The Ultimate Guide to Preventing and Curing Heart Disease with Diet and Supplements*, New York: HarperPaperbacks, 2000.

Childre, Doc Lew, *Freeze Frame*, Boulder Creek, CA: Planetary Publications, 1994.

Cloud, Dr. Henry, *Changes that Heal: How to Understand Your Past to Ensure a Healthier Future*, Grand Rapids, MI: Zondervan Publishing House, 1996.

Dale, Cyndi, *Attracting Your Perfect Body through the Chakras*, Berkeley, CA: The Crossing Press, 2006.

Diamond, John, M.D., *Your Body Doesn't Lie*, New York: Warner Books, 1989.

Gerber, Richard, M.D., *A Practical Guide to Vibrational Medicine*, New York: Perennial Currents, 2001.

Hay, Louise, *You Can Heal Your Life*, Carlsbad, CA: Hay House, 1999.

Jacka, Judy, N.D., *The Vivaxix Connection*, Charlottesville, VA: Hampton Roads Publishing Company, 2000.

Johnson, Steven, *Mind Wide Open: Your Brain and the Neuroscience of Everyday Life*, New York: Scribner, 2004.

Kabat-Zinn, Jon, Ph.D., *Full Catastrophe Living*, New York: Delta Trade Paperbacks, 1990.

Lowry, Lois, *The Giver*, New York: Laurel-Leaf Books, 1993.

Null, Gary, Ph.D., *The Clinician's Handbook of Natural Healing*, New York: Kensington Books, 1997.

Ornish, Dean, M.D., *Reversing Heart Disease*, New York: Ballantine Books, 1990.

Pert, Candace, Ph.D., *Molecules of Emotion*, New York: Scribner, 1999.

Schwarzbein, Diana, M.D., *The Shwarzbein Principle II*, Deerfield, FL: Health Communications, Inc., 2002.

Taylor, Cathryn L., M.A., *The Inner Child Workbook*, New York: Jeremy P. Tarcher/Putnam, 1991.

Whitaker, Julian M., M.D. *Reversing Heart Disease*, New York: Warner Books, 2002.

Power

Campbell, Joseph, and Moyers, Bill, *The Power of Myth*, New York: Doubleday, 1988.

Cooper, Susan, *The Dark Is Rising*, New York: Aladdin Paperbacks, 1973. (As well as the rest of The Dark is Rising series.)

Emoto, Masaru, *The True Power of Water*, Hillsboro, OR: Beyond Words, 2005.

Gardner, Laurence, *Genesis of the Grail Kings*, Gloucester, MA: Fair Winds Press, 2002.

Hawkins, David, *Power versus Force: The Hidden Determinants of Human Behavior*, Carlsbad, CA: Hay House, 2002.

Hawkins, David, *Transcending the Levels of Consciousness*, Sedona, AZ: Veritas, 2005.

Hunbatz, Men, *The Secrets of Mayan Science/Religion*, Santa Fe, NM: Bear & Company, 1990.

Mails, Thomas, *Fools Crows Wisdom & Power*, Tulsa, OK: Council Oaks Books, 1991.

Morgan, Marlo, *Mutant Message Down Under*, Lees Summit, MO: MM Co., 1991.

Myss, Carolyn, Ph.D., *Invisible Acts of Power: Personal Choices that Create Miracles*, New York: Free Press, 2004.

Tolle, Eckhart, *The Power of Now*, Novato, CA and Vancouver, BC, CAN: New World Library and Namaste Publishing, 1999.

Trungpa, Choygam, *The Sacred Path of the Warrior*, Boston: Shambala, 1984.

Webster, Richard, *Spirit Guides and Angel Guardians*, St. Paul, MN: Llewellyn Publications, 1998.

Imagination

Attanasio, A.A., *The Serpent and the Grail*, New York: Harper Prism, 1999.

Atwater, P.M.H., *Future Memory*, Charlottesville, VA: Hampton Roads, 1999.

Bradley, Marion Zimmer, *The Mists of Avalon*, New York: Random House, 1982.

Castaneda, Carlos, *A Separate Reality*, New York: Pocket Books, 1971.

Eliade, Mircea, *Shamanism: Archaic Techniques of Ecstasy*, Princeton, NJ: Bollingen Foundation, 1964.

Kaku, Michio, Ph.D., *Hyperspace: A Scientific Odyssey Through Parallel Universes*, New York: Anchor, 1995.

Harman, Willis, Ph.D., and Rheingold, Howard, *Higher Creativity*, New York: The Putnam Publishing Group, 1984.

Hosseini, Khaled, *The Kite Runner*, New York: Riverhead Books, 2003.

Lackey, Mercedes, *The Fairy Godmother*, New York: Luna Books, 2004.

Newton, Michael, Ph.D., *Journey of Souls*, St. Paul, MN: Llewellyn Publications, 1994.

Perkins, John, *The World As You Dream It*, Rochester, VT: Destiny Books, 1994.

Popescu, Petru, *Amazon Beaming*, New York: Penguin Books, 1991.

Skully, Nicki, *The Golden Cauldron: Shamanic Journeys on the Path of Wisdom & Power*, Rochester, VT: Bear & Company, 1991.

Villoldo, Alberto, Ph.D., *Shaman, Healer, Sage*, New York: Harmony, 2000.

Zukav, Gary, *The Dancing Wu Li Masters*, New York: Bantam Books, 1979.

Divine

Brinkley, Dannion, *The Secrets of the Light*, Henderson, NV: HeartLight Productions, 2004.

Childre, Doc, and Martin, Howard, *The HeartMath Solution*, San Francisco: HarperSanFrancisco, 2000.

Chodron, Pema, *When Things Fall Apart*, Boston: Shambhala Publishers, 2002.

Cleary, Thomas, *The Taoist I Ching*, Boston: Shambhalla Publishers, 2002.

Cremo, Michael A., *Human Devolution: A Vedic Alternative to Darwin's Theory*, Badger, CA: Torchlight Publishing, 2003.

De Sainte Exupery, Antoine, *The Little Prince*, New York: Harcourt, Inc., 1943.

Gallico, Paul, *The Snow Goose*, New York: Alfred A. Knopf, 2000.

Kelsey, Morton, *Healing & Christianity*, Minneapolis, MN: Augsburg Press, 1995.

Lewis, C.S., *The Lion, The Witch and the Wardrobe*, New York: Harper Trophy, 1950. (As well as the Chronicles of Narnia series.)

Rilke, Rainer Maria, *Letters to a Young Poet: The Possibility of Being*, New York: MJF Books, 2000.

Shealy, C. Norman, M.D., *Sacred Healing: The Curing Power of Energy & Spirituality*, Lanham, MD: Element Books Ltd., 1999.

Stepanek, Mattie, J.T., *Journey Through Heartsongs*, New York: Hyperion, 2001.

Walsch, Neale Donald, *Tomorrow's God: Our Greatest Spiritual Challenge*, New York: Atria, 2004.

Additional Resources:

Brain Sync audio programs and CDs. Spirituality series. www.brainsync.com.

Endnotes

Introduction

1. Waltari, Mika, *A Nail Merchant at Nightfall* (New York: G.P. Putnam's Sons, 1954), p. 9.

Chapter One

1. Ripp, James M., M.D., *Heart Disease for Dummies* (Hoboken, NJ: Wiley Publishing, 2004), p.11.

2. Ibid, p.8.

3. Pearsall, Paul, Ph.D., *The Heart's Code* (New York: Broadway Books, 1998), p. 55.

4. McCraty, Rollin, Ph.D., *The Energetic Heart* (Boulder Creek, CA: HeartMath Institute Research Center, 2003), p.1.

5. McCraty, Rollin, Ph.D., Atkinson, Mike, and Tomasino, Dana, *Science of the Heart* (Boulder Creek, CA: HeartMath Institute Research Center, 2001).

6. McCraty, Rollin, Ph.D., *The Energetic Heart*, p. 1.

7. Bunzel, B., et al, "Does Changing the Heart Mean Changing Personality? A Retrospective Inquiry on 47 Heart Transplant Patients," *Quality of Life Research*, Vol. 1 (1992): pp. 251–256.

8. Rein, G., and McCraty, R., "Modulation of DNA by Coherent Heart Frequencies." Proceedings of the 3rd Annual Conference of the

International Society for the Study of Subtle Energies and Energy
Medicine, Monterey, CA, June 1993.

9. McCraty, Rollin, Ph.D., *The Energetic Heart*, p. 14.

Chapter Two

1. Cortis, Bruno, M.D., *Heart & Soul: A Psychological and Spiritual Guide to Healing Heart Disease* (New York: Villard Books, 1995), pp. 4–5; Ornish, Dean, M.D., *Dr. Dean Ornish's Program for Reversing Heart Disease* (New York: Ballantine Books, 1990), p. 1; Ripp, James M., M.D., *Heart Disease for Dummies* (Hoboken, NJ: Wiley Publishing, 2004), pp. 8, 10; Cortis, Bruno, M.D., *Heart & Soul*, p. 10; Simon, Harvey B., M.D., *Conquering Heart Disease* (New York: Little, Brown and Company, 1994), p. 3; Simon, p. 37; Ripp, p. 97.

2. Underwood, Anne, "The Good Heart," in *Newsweek* (October 3, 2005): p. 50.

3. Ibid, p. 51.

4. Ibid, p. 51.

5. His Holiness the Dalai Lama, *The Good Heart* (Boston: Wisdom Publications, 1996), p. 112.

6. Zukav, Gary, *The Seat of the Soul* (New York: Free Press, 1990), p. 94.

7. Gerber, Richard, M.D., *Vibrational Medicine* (Sante Fe: Bear & Company, 1988), p. 376.

8. Ibid, pp. 376–377.

9. Men, Hunbatz, *Secrets of Mayan Science/Religion* (Santa Fe: Bear & Company, 1990), p. 126.

10. Corbin, Henry, *Creative Imagination in the Sufism of Ibn Arabi*, trans. Ralph Manheim (Princeton, NJ: Princeton University Press, 1969), pp. 221–36.

11. McCraty, Rollin, Ph.D., *The Appreciative Heart* (Boulder Creek, CA: HeartMath Institute Research Center, 2003), pp. 1–3.

12. Ibid, pp. 9–10.

13. McCraty, Rollin, Ph.D., *The Energetic Heart*, p. 11.

14. McCraty, Rollin, Ph.D., *The Appreciative Heart*, pp. 6–8.

15. Ibid, pp. 5–8.

16. McTaggart, Lynne, *The Field* (New York: Harper Perennial, 2002), p. 23.

17. Emoto, M., "Healing with Water," in *Journal of Alternative and Complementary Medicine* 10, no. 1 (2004):19–21.

18. McCraty, Rollin, Ph.D., *The Energetic Heart*, p. 3.

19, Ibid, p. 2.

20. James L. Oschman, *Energy Medicine* (New York: Churchill Livingstone, 2000), p. 18.

21. Gerber, Richard, M.D., *A Practical Guide to Vibrational Medicine* (New York: HarperCollins Publishers, 2000), p. 274.

Chapter Three

1. Ornish, Dean, M.D., *Reversing Heart Disease* (New York: Ballantine Books, 1990) p. 81.

2. Brett, AS, "Treating Hypercholesterolemia: How Should Practicing Physicians Interpret the Published Data for Patients?" in *New England Journal of Medicine* 321 (1989): 676–80.

3. Leaf, A., "Management of Hypercholesterolemia," in *New England Journal of Medicine* 321 (1989): 680–83.

4. Challem, Jack, *The Inflammation Syndrome* (Hoboken, NJ: John Wiley & Sons, 2003), p. 15.

5. Simon, Harvey B., M.D., *Conquering Heart Disease* (New York: Little, Brown & Company, 1994), p. 19.

6. Challem, Jack, *The Inflammation Syndrome*, p. 42.

7. Page, J., and Henry, D., "Consumption of NSAIDS and the Development of Congestive Heart Failure in Elderly Patients: An Underrecognized Public Health Problem" in *Archives of Internal Medicine* 160 (2000): 777–784.

8. Ornish, Dean, M.D., *Reversing Heart Disease*, p. 57.

9. Challem, Jack, *The Inflammation Syndrome*, p. 55.

10. Cutler JA, MacMahon SW, and Furberg CD, "Controlled Clinical Trials of Drug Treatment for Hypertension" in *Hypertension* 13, suppl. I (1989): I36–I44.

11. Cortis, Bruno, M.D., *Heart & Soul*, p. 92.

12. Ibid, p. 66.

13. Ornish, Dean, M.D., *Reversing Heart Disease*, pp. 18–19.

14. Ibid, p. 102.

15. House JS, Robbins C, and Metzner HL, "The Association of Social Relationships and Activities with Mortality: Prospective Evidence from the Tecumseh Community Health Study" in *American Journal of Epidemiology* 116, no. 1 (1982): 123–40.

16. Deanfield, JE, and Selwyn, AP, "Character and Causes of Transient Myocardial Ischemia During Daily Life: Implications for Treatments

of Patients with Coronary Disease." in *Lancet* 8410, no. 2 (1984):
1001–1005.

17. Green, Cindy L., Ph.D., et al, "Prayer, Noetic Studies Feasible: Results
Indicate Benefit to Heart Patients" (paper, Duke University Medical
Center, Durham, NC, October 2001), as published in the Science Blog,
copyright 2004, http://www.scienceblog.com/community/older/2001
/B/200111913.html, accessed August, 2006.

Chapter Four

1. Richard, Gerber, M.D., *Vibrational Medicine*, p. 111.
2. Bruyere, Rosalyn, *Wheels of Light* (Sierra Madre, CA: Bon Productions,
1989), pp. 247–259.
3. Jacobson, Theodore A., and Parentani, Renaud, "An Echo of Black
Holes," in *Scientific American* 293, no. 6 (December 2005): 69–75.
4. Underwood, Anne, "The Good Heart," p. 52.
5. Ibid, p. 51.

Chapter Five

1. McCraty, Rollin, Ph.D., Atkinson, Mike, and Bradley, Raymond
Trevor, Ph.D., "The Electrophysiological Evidence of Intuition: Part 2.
A System-Wide Process?" in *Journal of Alternative and Complementary
Medicine* 10, no. 2 (2004): 325–336. Also available in abstract form
through the HeartMath Research Center at the Institute of HeartMath.

Chapter Ten

1. Payne, Robert, *The Life and Death of Mahatma Gandhi* (New York:
Konecky & Konecky, 1969), p. 372.
2. Matthew 21: 21.

Index

standing waveforms, 37
star beings, 206, 207
star element, 192–193
statin drugs. *See* cholesterol lowering drugs
stenosis, 88t
stone beings, 206
stone element, 191
stones and rocks, properties of, 181
Street of Hope, 34
strep infections, 97
stress
    cardiovascular disease and, 24–25
    impact on adrenaline levels, 77
    impact on blood flow, 68
    strokes, 24, 50–51, 92t, 93t
    strongholds, 81, 193–195
Suarez, Edward, 24
sudden cardiac arrest, 49, 87t, 94t
supernatural strength. *See* power pathway
supplements, primary disease chakra
    and, 187–188
surgery, 178–179
swimming, benefits of, 184
symbology
    of chakras, 120
    healing with, 127–131
symbology issues, auric bands and, 200
symbols, using, 124
sympathy
    described, 104
    types of, 107–111

tachyons, 10, 35
tennis/racquetball, 184
tenth chakra
    about, 94–95t, 111
    described, 74t
    physiological location of, 76t
    relationship with nature and
        environment, 181–182
thalamus, and the heart, 8
theory of relativity. *See* "New Science"
third chakra
    about, 108–109
    chronic heart failure, 90t
    described, 73t
    physiological location of, 76t
thrombosis, chronic heart failure, 90t
thyroid, and heart palpitations, 147
Tibetan Buddhism, view of the heart, 26
time and space energy factors, 38–39
time travel, 204
tonal differences, in the major chakras, 73
tones
    of chakras, 120
    of whole notes, 131–132

toning, using, 124
transformation, of a contract or
    interference, 152
transmission, described, 104
transpersonal process, 152–153
triglycerides, 55
twelfth chakra
    about, 96t
    described, 74t
    physiological location of, 76t
twelve-chakra healing system, x
twelve spiritual gates, 233, 235t

unbonding exercise, 188–189
the unconscious, and the Middle
    Heart, 173–174

valvular disease
    about, 48
    childhood illness and, 94t
    first chakra and, 88t, 89t
    personal boundaries and, 95t
    resistance and, 174
    tissue disorders and, 96t
varicose veins, 52, 87t, 94t
vascular diseases, 96
vasculitis, 51, 88t
venous incompetence, 51, 93t
venous thrombosis, 51–52, 88t
verbal sympathy, 109
very low-density lipoproteins (VLDLs), 55
vibration, 36–37
    See also frequency
vibrational disorders, 62
vibrational healing, overview, 117–120
Vibrational Medicine (Gerber), 27, 72
virtues, 214, 220
viruses, outside causes of, 97
visual sympathy, 109–110
Vivaxis, 138–139, 200–201
vulnerability. *See* divine pathway

wakefulness, 26
walking, benefits of, 183
water beings, 206
water cleansing, 183
water element, 190
weightlifting, benefits of, 184
white wash, 155
white zone, 205
wholeness, intention to produce, 175
Wittstein, Ilan, 77
wood beings, 207
wood element, 191

yoga, benefits of, 184

Zukav, Gary, 26